THE

Me

I KNEW

I COULD BE

THE
Me
I KNEW
I COULD BE

Crystal Phillips

ST. MARTIN'S GRIFFIN
NEW YORK

For information, address
St. Martin's Press, 175 Fifth Avenue, New York, N.Y. 10010.

www.stmartins.com

Design by Mary A. Wirth

Library of Congress Cataloging-in-Publication Data

Phillips, Crystal.
    The me I knew I could be : one woman's journey from 292 pounds to
peace, happiness, and healthy living / Crystal Phillips.
        p. cm.
    Includes bibliographical references.
    ISBN 0-312-25226-9 (hc)
    ISBN 0-312-27076-3 (pbk)
    1. Phillips, Crystal. 2. Eating disorders. 3. Weight loss. 4. Body image.
5. Health. I. Title.

RC552.E18 P48 2001
616.85'26'0092—dc21
[B]
                                                                    00-047046

10 9 8 7 6 5 4

Dedicated In Loving Memory

My brother Kevin Phillips—his fighting spirit to live life to the fullest even toward the end has taught me to never live in fear and to be grateful for one's good health. Through him I have learned courage.

My aunt Delores Goosby—I'm grateful for our long talks on the phone while I was away in college. I felt alone and disconnected, but you were my bridge guiding me back to my mother.

My sister Angela Phillips—your creative talents and bright mind have given me the courage to soar to higher levels in my journey to learn more about myself and find balance so that I can help others.

CONTENTS

ACKNOWLEDGMENTS

I am grateful for each day God has given me and for blessing me with good health. I'm blessed to have such wonderful and supportive parents, Dr. Roy and Vira Phillips. Dad, the hardest-working man I know, thanks for always being my rock of faith and for always showing me by example how to take the high road. Mom, I love you for always being my voice of reason and comfort. I don't know what I'd do without you. I thank my brother Roy Phillips, Jr., for being in my corner and giving sound exercise advice. I thank my sister-in-law Deborah Phillips for all of your support. I thank God for my sister Kelley for being my friend and my mirror of beauty from the inside out. I am thankful for my little brothers and sister, Duane, Alex, and April. Thank you, Aunt Vernell, for showing me how to keep going on when times get rough. Much love to Uncle Andrew and Aunt Josephine for always remembering me on my birthday.

I am grateful for the friends who have stuck by me through

thick and thin: Yvette Hatcher, Charlotte Bullock, Katrina Robinson, Michael Bracey, Kuji, and Alfred Wesson who keeps me honest.

Special thanks to: Alan Leo for his words of wisdom and great photography; Karen Hiter for her beautiful artistry in make-up.

Thanks to Dr. Simpler, Dr. Sortisio, and Dr. Steiner for keeping me healthy. I thank Dr. Bernetta George for your kindness and care of my brother Kevin. Dr. Micheal Zollicoffer, thanks for always supporting me and my products. Much thanks and gratitude to my literary agent, Virginia Amos, for tracking me down after reading my story in *Ebony* magazine. I am grateful to you for never selling me short and for holding my hand through all the writing and rewrites. You've been a great friend and you're simply the best! Thanks to Nicole Walker for the wonderful *Ebony* magazine article, to Kelly Starling for the "Bookshelf" review, and many thanks to Susan Taylor. Deborah Gregory of *Essence*, the first magazine to share my story and the first to represent the beauty of all my sisters. Enormous thanks to *Fitness* and *Living Fit* magazines for publishing my story, as well as to *The Baltimore Sun*. I'm grateful to the Radio One family 95.9 and 92Q for allowing me to share my story with your listeners. Much gratitude to WWRL (1600) in New York. I thank WBAL-TV, WJZ, and WMAR television stations.

I am especially grateful to Jennifer Enderlin, my editor, who made my dreams come true. Thank you for believing in my story and me and for coming up with a fantastic book title.

Thanks to Denise Carpenter, Noreen Callahan, Cliff Denby, Patrick Emery, the Towson YMCA, The Columbia Gym, and my personal trainer, my dog Heru.

Finally, last but not least, I want to thank the lady who inspired me to do the work from within, Oprah Winfrey.

INTRODUCTION

*I*n the words of my favorite jazz artist, Dianne Reeves, "I just want to testify." Six years ago, I weighed almost three hundred pounds. Constant bingeing left a legacy of depression that made getting out of bed—much less out of the house—a daily struggle. My legs were so fat that my inner thighs were raw and bleeding by the end of the day. The ache in my joints and back never went away. Walking from my apartment to my car, or from my car to an appointment, or from my car to the grocery store was exhausting. But it didn't stop me from getting just one more package of steaks or just one more quart of ice cream. I spent money on food like an alcoholic does on liquor or a drug addict on a fix. I was totally out of control. There was no "me." There was just a fat, hulking body pretending to be a person with hopes and dreams and of a tomorrow. I was no longer a human being but an object to ridicule, abuse, and humiliate. And I didn't even have to walk out my front door—I did that all to myself.

I wanted to end my life.

I made a choice to live instead. I stopped looking to the outside and started looking within for the miracle God creates in all of us. I didn't lose weight for my parents or to get a man. I didn't lose weight for a job or a high school reunion or a wedding or because I wanted to be a certain size. I lost weight because I wanted to love myself again.

I lost 157 pounds, nine dress sizes, two shoe sizes, three bra sizes, two ring sizes, and one hat size. In return, I gained my dignity, my freedom, my spirit, and my life.

There is no magic plan here, so don't go skipping pages looking for something you can cut out and paste up on your refrigerator door. Read everything. Stick with me and you will learn why you eat when you aren't hungry, why you may attract negative forces in your life, why a strong foundation will keep you motivated, why exercise is fun, why you need to have a WAR bag, why honesty is always the best policy, and why you need to stop dieting.

I don't promise easiness or quickness but I do promise a new way of life that can bring you health and happiness if you just let it happen. How do I know this can work for you? Because it worked for me. I am not a TV personality or a model. I do not have a chef or lots of time on my hands. I work at my job and my life every day. I have ups and downs and get frustrated. I laugh and cry. I am just another sister trying to get by.

I am here with you.

THE
Me
I KNEW
I COULD BE

1

ONE LAST TIME

*I*t's December 31, 1994. My brother is dead, my Aunt Delores is dead, and my parents have lost their house in a hurricane. I, Crystal, have had major surgery and have left my husband. All I want to do now is pick up the pieces of my life and put them back together. But how can I, when there is nothing? I am thirty-four years old, and despite weighing 245 pounds, I am totally empty inside. I have starved off fifty pounds, but it is just a matter of time before the scale reaches three hundred pounds again. I feel old, fat, and miserable. I simply want to die.

A girlfriend has invited me to go to church with her for a New Year's Eve service. The part of me hanging on to one last thread of hope agrees to go. I struggle into a too-tight skirt and take my place. I am afraid my waistband will open if I walk forward to the altar and kneel to pray, so I stay in my seat and wait. I don't remember much about the sermon or the service or the ride home. I just know that something is different. I take a long hard look at myself in the mirror and then get down on my knees. I surrender to God's power and to his love and make a commitment—to me.

I'm not tired or angry or even hungry. I move to the TV and pick up a tape of an old *Oprah Winfrey Show*. Oprah is talking about her second dramatic weight loss and challenging her viewing audience to embark on a journey of self-discovery by feeling the feelings and letting them go. I wasn't ready for this message the first time I heard it and I'm not sure I am ready this time. I'm terrified. *But what about the commitment I just made?* Aren't I worth it?

2

MOTOWN—MOTORTOWN "CHILDHOOD"

I can remember when food was *not* an issue for me. I was about four years old and spent most of my time running just to keep up with my older brothers. I didn't have a weight problem as a child. Back then, Mama had to call me more than once to come in to eat lunch or dinner. I was always in a hurry to get back outside to play. I loved being a tomboy—climbing trees, running relay races, and wrestling with the boys. I didn't play with the girls in my neighborhood much because they never wanted to roughhouse around and were afraid to get their dresses dirty. But not me. At birthday parties I was the one who was always out on the dance floor, the first ready to get the party started. I was known as the roadrunner baby. I ate quickly and had to be bribed to finish my meals 'cause I could hear I was missing out on all the fun outside. Sometimes Mom would bribe me with the promise of a Good Humor ice cream bar if I would just finish my dinner.

Our family was really pretty average. I had two older brothers, Mom was a housewife, and Dad was a high school math/science teacher. But Dad also had great ambitions—every spare minute and every summer were spent in pursuit of more education. He would eventually get both his Master's and Ph.D. degrees.

Mom was my best friend. Whenever she had the car keys, I knew we were going shopping at Hudson's or the secondhand store. I loved these trips, when Mom was all mine, not distracted by Roy, Junior, or Kevin.

We could get away with murder when Mom wasn't around because Dad was always preoccupied with studying for school. The three of us would sneak away and watch "The Little Rascals" and "The Three Stooges" on TV—shows forbidden because of the negative racial stereotypes and violence. As long as we didn't disturb him too much, Dad was a real pushover. I think sometimes he felt guilty for not spending a lot of his free time with us, so he would give us the loose change in his pocket and we would run to the corner store for penny candy.

Some Saturdays when Dad took me to run errands with him, he would get so caught up talking business with the endless business friends we'd cross paths with that when it was time to leave I'd feel faint from hunger. All I had to do was keep pulling his coat jacket, telling him I was hungry, and he'd absentmindedly pat me on the head and give me money to fetch a hot dog and a bag of potato chips for us to share. I loved it when Dad picked me up because I could never get junk food out of Mom. With Mom, we always left on time and I'd usually have something like leftovers waiting for me to eat at home.

The summer I was five, Dad was away working on his graduate degree, and my Aunt Delores came to live with us. My brothers and I were all just eleven months apart and a real handful for Mom.

I loved to dance and would spend rainy summer days with Detroit's number-one radio station, WCHB, listening to Martha Jean the Queen playing all the Motown hits. I would dance for hours in front of a floor-length mirror. I'd lose track of time and all my surroundings when I danced. I felt safe and secure in my own little world—and then Mom decided to enroll me in my first ballet class.

Lordy, I was so excited I couldn't sleep the night before. I kept getting out of bed to look at my leotards, tights, tap shoes, and pink ballet slippers. That Saturday morning, before class started, Mom told me to pay close attention to the instructor. No need to worry about me. I always made sure I was the first one on the dance floor so I could look at my reflection in the enormous wall-length mirror and practice my dance steps. There were lots of distractions, especially when some of the little girls left crying because it was too hard. I was happy when they didn't come back because the overcrowded class grew smaller and smaller and I finally had room to express myself and move to my heart's content. Without fail, after every class, one of the mothers would ask Mom where I had taken dance lessons before coming to that studio. Mom, with pride and enthusiasm, would say that this was my first time taking lessons and the other mothers would look at her in disbelief. I was so happy!

It wasn't until a few weeks later that the instructor's attitude toward me began to change. She suddenly insisted that I move to the back. I thought maybe she was having everyone take turns being in the front row, but no one else was ever asked to move to the back. Whenever I asked to be in the front row or went to the front on my own, the instructor would give me an irritated look and then impatiently pull me to the back. Some of the class depended on me to remember the routines, so they continued to look to the back to see what I was doing. The instructor would get angry and yell for them to look to the front and to her for cues. The class followed suit and began treating me badly. The girls stopped sharing their snacks and started calling me ugly while they tossed their long wavy hair from side to side. The longer I stood in the back of the room, the more I noticed how different I looked from everyone else. It only took a few more weeks for me to give up.

The dance studio was owned by an African-American woman and all the instructors and students were African-American, but I was the only one with dark skin and two teaspoons of kinky hair. I began to feel unattractive and like I didn't belong, especially when I was teased about not having long Shirley Temple curls. When I looked in the mirror I was beginning NOT to like what was staring back at me. I wanted to look like the girls in my dance class who looked "good enough" to dance in the front row. I wanted long flowing hair and light skin.

As time went on, my joy in dance began to fade. It became a chore for Mom to get me excited and ready for my Saturday ballet class. Mom noticed the change in my behavior and stayed behind to watch rehearsal. She noticed my location in the back row and how mean the instructor was toward me, and pulled me out of that dance studio that very day. As she drove home, with fury in her eyes, she vowed to find another dance studio where they would appreciate a talented dancer. She also said that the studio had lost out on a great student who had a lot to offer. I'll never forget how at the next light Mom looked me straight in the eye, took my hand and told me I was beautiful, smart, and talented, and then kissed my forehead. As we drove off I looked at my reflection in the window and studied my dark skin and short kinky hair. But I had begun to doubt all those things my mother was so sure of.

In the summer of 1968, Mom asked Dad to take my brothers and me to California to visit his parents. She had never been away from us and needed a break from the daily rigors of three active children. I remember my brothers jumping up and down for joy.

I, on the other hand, was not with the program. Going to California was like going to prison. My grandfather's second wife never had any children of her own and was overly protective, never wanting to let us out of her sight. Since the Watts riots had occurred three years previous, and the recent assassinations of Martin Luther King and Robert F. Kennedy, we probably wouldn't even be allowed to look out the window. I knew I would be stuck in the house with Grandma. And all summer long Grandma would try to interest me in learning to crochet.

But I also envisioned myself having fun riding around in my cousin's Mustang convertible looking at the famous big white Hollywood sign that I saw in all the movies and magazines. I wanted to take a tour of the stars' homes, and go to the ocean to play in the salt water. Instead I was going to be stuck learning to crochet and getting sick watching Grandmother chew on her tobacco and spit into her old tin coffee can. Daytime soap operas were my grandmother's other passion. Knowing Dad, he would take off to visit old friends and my brothers and I would have to sit and watch those miserable old "soaps" with Grandma. Like always, I'd daydream to make the time pass, and imagine what we were going to have for dinner. But Grandma wasn't a very good cook so that daydream had some holes in it. The only things she did cook really well were Seven-Up cake, homemade rolls, and roast beef.

Before leaving for California, I asked Mom if I could stay home with her for the summer. "No" she soothed me, "you'll have a good time." Dad reminded me that we would go to Disneyland and spend the whole day enjoying rides and games. I was still not thrilled about our journey west. Everyone else but me started counting down the days until our cross-country trip.

A few days before we left, Mom sat me down and taught me to style my hair on my own. I was wearing a ponytail hairpiece that matched my own coarse hair. For years, people thought it was my hair. Although Mom always wore her hair in a short natural cut, she couldn't convince me to do the same. I wore my hair natural at the time, but I no longer wanted short hair. Mom decided to buy this hairpiece for me, realizing the politics of hair in our society and hoping to raise my self-esteem after the incident at the dance studio. Each time Mom bought a new ponytail for me, she'd secure it into my hair with a rubber band and leave the ponytail loose. Then she'd tell me to go play. I'd ask her to put on Ike and Tina Turner's "Proud Mary" and I'd dance around shaking my hair like Tina Turner until I was dripping with sweat and my pony-tail piece was as kinky as my own hair. The shower was the next stop, to wash my dusty hair. Afterward Mom would towel dry my hair, put Brylcreem on it, and I'd have a fresh, fluffy braid or twisted pigtails dangling to my shoulders.

Mom spent hours with me showing me what took only minutes for her to do. While she helped me with my lopsided ponytail, she casually but carefully instructed me to lock all bathroom and bed-room doors while dressing or undressing in California. Mom also instructed me to lock the bathroom door while I bathed and always to wear my robe with my pajamas. She said, very gently and in a voice designed not to scare me, "Grandpa has a tendency to walk in on women without warning." She said he had done this to her the last time we visited, so I was to be careful and follow her instructions. She reassured me, "He probably won't ever walk in on you, but if he does, you scream and tell somebody right away."

I agreed and didn't think anything more about it. It just all sounded silly to me.

That first evening in California, after my brothers had show-ered, I remembered what Mom told me and tried to lock the bath-room door, but the lock was not working. I thought since Grandpa saw me going into the bathroom, he would not come in, especially after he warned me the water might be a little cool since Roy, Jr., and Kevin had taken long showers. I hadn't developed yet and thought to myself, "There's nothing here for Grandpa to see." My final thought put my mind at ease and I slipped into a tub filled with Mr. Bubbles.

Just as I started washing my face, the bathroom door opened. Grandpa stood there, quickly trying to scan my body. He had a look of fascination in his eyes that I'll never forget. I screamed at the top of my lungs as Grandpa calmly left. I jumped out of the tub, covering myself, then quickly put on my pajamas. I was shocked, afraid, embarrassed, angry, and sorry all at once. I was shocked he would do this to his own granddaughter. I felt sorry for Dad for having this man as a father. Dad adored his father and talked about him as if he were a saint. I was afraid to tell because I didn't think Dad would believe me, and I didn't want a big confrontation between the two of them if he did believe me. I was angry with Mom for not letting me stay home with her and because nobody came to my rescue when I screamed. But then I realized I had placed the facecloth tightly over my mouth when I screamed.

I lay awake for hours that night, fearful Grandpa would try to sneak into my room while I slept. I got up and pushed my heavy suitcase against the door. I prayed to God for most of the night never to let my breasts develop or let me have a menstrual cycle so I could never have babies or develop pubic hair. In the wee hours of the morning, I finally drifted off.

I nearly jumped out of my skin when I heard a loud knock on my bedroom door. Roy, Jr., and Kevin were yelling for me to hurry and get dressed because Dad was taking us to Disneyland.

The lines were too long, the day too hot, and I was too tired and hungry to enjoy anything. By the time noon came, my little body was drained and I was feeling sick. Dad bought us snowballs to cool us down and to quench our thirst. He gave me pineapple instead of lemon, which made me even sicker. I put my head on the picnic table, waiting for Dad to bring back our hamburgers and fries. He was standing in another long line for the food. I was fast asleep before he ever came back.

The smell of roast beef, mashed potatoes, string beans, and homemade rolls brought me back to life. We were back at Grandpa's house and my stomach started to knot up again. After I washed up, I went out to the table feeling like I could eat the whole meal myself. Everyone catered to my every need, even Roy, Jr., and Kevin. I loved it and played it for all it was worth. When it was time for us to take our evening bath, I claimed that maybe I shouldn't take a bath at night. I lied and said the night air after bathing was making me sick. Grandma told me to take my baths in the morning from here on out. I smiled faintly, trying to look as pitiful as I could. I was happy that I could now bathe after Grandpa left for work.

That night Grandma piled so many quilts on me that I thought I would suffocate from the heat. I took all the quilts off after she closed my bedroom door. I could overhear Grandpa and Grandma talking while watching TV. They were talking about some movie star that had recently put on a lot of weight. The last thing I remember hearing Grandpa say was something about how unattractive fat made a woman. That night I dreamed that Grandpa had managed to open my bedroom door. He was reaching to take the heavy quilts off me to look at my body. By the time he reached the last quilt, I woke up and proudly revealed my three-hundred-pound naked body. I watched his mouth drop open and his face turn to horror as he ran out of the room screaming at the top of his lungs.

Dad rescued us the next afternoon by taking us to our aunt's house for a barbecue. I was starting to get hooked on the daytime soap operas and asked Grandma to brief me on what happened when we returned. She happily agreed.

Before the car reached my auntie's house, we could hear the sounds of Motown and smell the barbecued ribs in the air. Her carefully manicured backyard held rows of picnic tables full of strangers. I wished that Mom was here, or better yet, I was back home with her. Dad started introducing us around, telling us how we were related to each man, woman, and child. Kevin was sharing a story with one of our uncles on how he and Roy, Jr., had met Gladys Knight when they were handing out campaign flyers at a polling place. I got bored and decided to wander around to see what we were going to eat.

I walked over to check out the meat table. There were at least six cases of smoked ribs, plates of catfish, grilled porterhouse steaks, grilled hamburgers, hot dogs, and red-hot sausage links. The vegetable table had fried okra, corn on the cob, cole slaw, potato salad, pickles, collard-and-turnip greens with ham hocks, tossed salads, and macaroni and cheese. On the bread table there were homemade rolls, hot-water corn bread, corn muffins, and regular white bread. Finally, my favorite, the dessert table—peach cobbler, apple cobbler, banana pudding, rum cake, pineapple upside-down cake, deep-dish apple pie, sweet potato pie, rice pudding, and a Jell-O fruit ring, with homemade ice cream on the way.

I was in hog heaven and went looking for a plate, but Auntie saw me first and gave me a big hug before I could make my way back to the table. Auntie said she knew we all must be starving staying over at Grandma's house and winked. "I know Grandma's cooking is probably different than what you're used to having at home. I even heard you were so sick from Grandma's cooking that you got sick at Disneyland." I didn't know where that rumor came from but I wasn't about to correct it. I just nodded my head and told her I was starving.

She took my plate and gave me everything I asked for without even saying, "Eat your vegetables first." She stood looking at me, smiling and watching me devour her tender barbecued ribs. When it was time for us to leave to go back to Grandpa's, I became fearful and said I wanted to stay with Auntie and her kids for the rest of our visit. But Dad said I'd hurt Grandma's feelings and that she would miss me when her daytime soaps came on. To stall for more time until I could think of a way to convince Dad, I claimed I was hungry. My aunts came to my rescue. They told Dad I was probably still hungry because I had been starving this whole time. I ate too much too fast, asking for more and more, pretending to be hungry, anything to keep from going back to my grandparents.

I took a final bite out of a porterhouse steak and lost it all. I had literally stuffed myself until my stomach couldn't hold any more. I had just had my first binge.

1972: 5'3"/140 lbs.

I was a frightened twelve-year-old girl living in a woman's body. Most people thought I was in my late teens or early twenties. When our next-door neighbor's son returned home from college, he asked me out for a date. I told him I was only twelve years old. He was extremely embarrassed and very apologetic.

In the seventh grade I was the tallest and the biggest girl in my class. I can remember being left out of slumber parties by my female classmates and harassed sexually by the boys. Sometimes Mom would dress me in beautiful African-influenced outfits—conservative sundresses with small matching head wraps—but I allowed my classmates to make me feel ashamed. They would call me the "African giraffe" and make fun of my height and dark complexion.

One time the principal, after seeing one of my outfits, directed me to sit in her office and then called my mother. She said I was distracting the other students and they could not focus on their work. Mom was furious at her. Ultimately I was sent home at lunchtime to change clothes. I dreaded going back to school because I knew by then the word had spread about the "African giraffe." I started turning to bigger portions of food for comfort and put on a few pounds. The extra weight made it difficult for me to dance en pointe (on toe) in my ballet class. My instructor and Mom thought I should lose some weight. My first diet!

Mom and I joined a weight-loss program together and slimmed down. I could enjoy my ballet lessons again and move without any restrictions, but being slim had its own problems. I was walking to my Saturday ballet class when I noticed my girlfriend's father stop pruning his bushes to watch me walk all the way down the street until I turned the corner. I lost count of the catcalls from passing cars as I stood at Livernois and Seven-Mile-Road. I was frightened. It was like being back at my grandfather's, except this time I had clothes on. If my clothes didn't keep men from looking at me, then something else would. I would be fat! No one ever seemed to bother the overweight girls in school or in ballet class. In fact, they seemed all but forgotten until they chose to make their presence known.

The next day I wore a sweater in ninety-degree weather to hide my body. Mom insisted that I take it off, but I didn't. Instead I grew resentful of her and started wearing baggy clothes to hide my hourglass figure. I knew I looked ridiculous but I never could seem to find the words to tell Mom what was troubling me. Mom had always been a wonderful mother, and I loved her dearly, but I was too ashamed to tell her that I hated my body or why I always locked my bedroom and bathroom doors while dressing and undressing and screamed at the top of my lungs whenever anyone knocked. When Mom tried to reach out to me, to ask questions or just to talk, I'd bite her head off and tell her to leave me alone. I'd feel so guilty afterward I'd punish and comfort myself at the same time by bingeing. It didn't take long to establish the pattern that would carry me into adulthood.

Food became my shield of armor from boys and my comfort when I'd overhear girls discussing weekend slumber parties, roller-skating parties, and other events they had enjoyed—events to which I had not been invited. I became moody and distant from my family. I had a younger sister now, Kelley, and I constantly fought with my two older brothers. I resented Mom and Dad for not protecting me from the things that I was unable to share with them. I simply did not know what to say or how to say it—and these were parents who loved and nurtured and wanted only the very best for me. The only way I knew how to deal with my feelings of shame, anger, fear, and loneliness was to eat.

1975: 5'4"/150 lbs.

I was fifteen-years old when Dad was offered an opportunity to advance his career. All of his years of going off to graduate school while we spent summers with Mom were starting to pay off. Dad worked nonstop. If he was home from work you could always find him reading in his study or writing. Dad was a wonderful provider, *but* the only time I interacted with him was when I had problems with homework—particularly math. My homework sessions with him were always short-lived when I couldn't grasp the concept of the math problems. I'd end up crying when I didn't comprehend what he was trying to teach me. The more impatient he grew with me, the more I cried. I felt stupid compared to Roy, Jr., and Kevin. They both were smart and could grasp all the abstract thinking of both math and science. After all the sobbing, erasing errors until holes appeared in my paper, Dad let me go to heal my hurt feelings. I'd have my stash of goodies hidden in my desk drawer in my bedroom to take away my throbbing headache and soothe my weary mind. Dad never once mentioned anything about my weight. Mom, on the other hand, was concerned.

Dad's new opportunity moved us from Detroit to the state of Washington: Mercer Island, right across the Puget Sound from Seattle. We were one of the few African-American families living on this affluent, predominantly white, island. Probably the only consolation was once standing in line at Safeway behind former basketball great Bill Russell. Mom had to tell me to close my mouth and stop staring up at him.

Before moving to the state of Washington, I made a silent promise (one of many) to God and myself that I would stop biting my nails and lose weight. My nails got better, but my weight stayed the same. I had just been accepted to Cass Technical High School in

Detroit and had not been happy when I learned we were moving to Washington. I was going to miss Aunt Delores, Aunt Vernell, and all my cousins.

I cried when I told my dance instructor and her daughter we were moving. I was teaching a few dance classes in the summer and was going to miss teaching the little five-year-olds tap and ballet. I loved them all and had helped one shy little girl with two teaspoons of kinky hair come out of her cocoon—just like I had wanted my first ballet teacher to do for me. The other girls began to include her for snacks and on the dance floor she began the slow process of feeling better about herself. Her parents were sorry to see me leave and I was sorry to go.

Moving to Mercer Island was a rude cultural awakening. I had always lived in mixed neighborhoods or all African-American neighborhoods. I had never been the only African-American anywhere. It was a chore trying to fit. I had immersed myself in ballet for so long I couldn't even show off with the latest dance moves from the home of Motown! My new classmates were disappointed. When I didn't join the jocks for sports, they were disappointed again. The "heads" (a great sixties word for anyone who smoked, drank, partied, did drugs, and/or promoted "free love") were disappointed when they realized I was not aligned with Angela Davis or Bobby Seale. When the bookworms saw I was just an average student and not a brain, they didn't know what to do with me either. It was a very lonely time.

1977: 5′4″ / 158 lbs.

In my senior year of high school, we moved again. I was seventeen. I was devastated when I learned we were moving to Omaha, Nebraska. If Washington State was bad, what in the world was Nebraska going to be like? Despite my misgivings, I finally settled in, and for the first time in a long while I developed good friendships with other girls. The senior prom was rapidly approaching, however, and I had no prospects in sight. By this time I was thankful if a tree looked my way. A week before the prom, a brother asked me to go with him and I said yes—to the prom and to a no-no relationship. Mom gently tried to warn me, especially on the evenings he promised to take me to the movies and never showed up. He would make the date for 7 P.M. and I would stand waiting for him at the window until 10 or 11 P.M.—like a dog waiting for his master to return. My parents were furious—at his behavior, but even more so with me for allowing it to happen. But I was determined to have a boyfriend at any cost. He did show up for the prom.

I graduated high school and stayed in Omaha to go to college. As I entered my last year in college, Dad was again offered a wonderful opportunity to advance his career. This time I was determined not to move. I had just landed a great part-time job, I was a senior, and my girlfriends and I had planned a trip out west after graduation. But most important, I was in love! Wow, no parents, no brothers, and no sister to interfere with my romance anymore. This was a dream come true. I settled and stayed in Nebraska while my family moved to Florida.

1983: 5'4"/165 lbs.

My boyfriend had grown tired of my Raggedy-Ann-doll ways. I lost count of the breaking up and making up and all the skinny minis I saw him with around town. Worst of all, I lost my full-time job. I had bought a house just two years before and the mortgage payments weren't going to stop just because I didn't have a paycheck coming in. I knew I could go to my parents but I was determined not to.

I was eating like a Nebraska Cornhusker and was beginning to look like one. Omaha was not big enough to escape the whispers of my unemployment or recent weight gain. I decided to rent my house and move to Baltimore, Maryland, where my brother Kevin was going to medical school (Johns Hopkins). At last I was making my own decision about moving. I was going to miss Omaha steaks, Goodrich ice cream, Valentino's pizza, and all the wonderful restaurants on Dodge Street. But hey, I heard Baltimore was famous for crab cakes!

3

THE WEDDING OR
THE NIGHTMARE?

*A*s much as I loved being in a big city, the move to Baltimore was hard and I found myself *needing* lots of food, and needing it fast. My bingeing took on epic proportions. And in May of 1985, my older brother, Kevin, graduated from Johns Hopkins Medical School and had finally come out to the family as a gay man. He was still family and we still loved him, but there was this virus that no one knew much about except that it was killing men in the gay community and we were afraid for Kevin.

In August of 1986, I was introduced to my husband, Steve, through a friend of my brother. I had already passed the two-hundred-pound mark, and my family and friends couldn't believe how much weight I was gaining. At this point I had given up on anyone ever being attracted to me because I was now officially a two-hundred-pounder. Who would want a woman weighing that much? I liked Steve, because he was honest and never tried to impress me with a lot of flattery or flashy clothes.

But I was not used to a man wanting to spend all of his time with me. Emotionally and physically unavailable men were more my style. I was used to breathing room.

One night when Steve kept asking me who I was seeing, I lost my temper and told him, "All the men in the neighborhood." Before I knew it, the left side of my face was burning. After it dawned on me that he had slapped me, I threw every ounce of my two-hundred-plus pounds on him and started beating him. His small car was rocking back and forth so fast that someone from my apartment complex called security.

I never told Mom or Dad because I knew exactly what they would say. "If a man hits you once, it won't be the last time." But I ignored all the warnings and the next three years turned into one long roller-coaster ride. I was as big a mess as Steve and I knew two messes together spelled disaster, but at least I was with someone. I knew this relationship was a reflection of how I felt about myself, but that wasn't enough to stop me.

Steve stuck to me like glue and I couldn't get rid of him. I'd explain to him that he needed to find his own friends and hobbies in addition to me, that I didn't think it was healthy for two people to spend so much time together. (Besides, I couldn't eat the way I wanted to around him and would get anxious about having all of my favorite binge foods.) But when I did manage to get rid of him, I'd see him with someone else and would start calling him to come over again. He'd accuse me of seeing other guys and started popping up at my door unannounced. There was never any other man at my house, but I guarantee you when I'd show up at his door without calling, there was always a sweet young thing around. I broke off with him so many times I couldn't believe he kept taking me back. For a change I wasn't the one sitting at home waiting for a phone call from the guy I was acting a hopeless fool over. This time I was in the driver's seat and it felt good! But one day my luck ran out and he gave me an ultimatum.

My self-esteem took a rapid dive when I said "I do" in 1989. Those weren't tears of joy at my wedding ceremony. I was crying because I wanted to throw my wedding bouquet in the toilet and run for the hills with a good divorce attorney. The day after our wedding, Steve took his former girlfriend, carrying his child, to have an abortion. The pressure was now on me for me to have lots of children, especially since I had demanded he choose between us during one of our many breakups,

I decided to get married because I felt it would be my last chance. "Who wants a woman weighing over two-hundred-pounds?" I thought. I still wasn't used to weighing so much. I've seen many beautiful women who weighed over two-hundred-pounds, but I couldn't ever seem to find the beauty in me. Steve and I had a silent contract with one another. I would accept him with all his faults and help him to become a citizen of this country, since he was not born in the United States. He was a hard worker and wanted to renovate a house for us. He had accepted me at two-hundred-plus pounds and I shared his dreams of having children someday, but not for at least a year or two or three or. Mom had told me long ago to enjoy being a newlywed and to get to know the man you married—and yourself—before having children. Bringing a child into the world is one of the greatest things a woman does in a lifetime, especially if you've chosen the right man to be by your side through the good and the bad times. But I was afraid to have children with Steve because I knew our marriage would not survive.

Before we married, I had these terrifying cold-sweat nightmares that I was pregnant with our fifth child. I was obese and miserable, and to make matters worse, the children never paid me any attention when I tried to discipline them. I would wake up screaming, "Please take the kids. I have to get some rest. I'm tired!"

I did everything in my power not to conceive. Since I couldn't take birth-control pills because of my uterine fibroids, I used at least three methods of birth control each time we were intimate. He knew I didn't want children right now, but he kept pressuring me nonstop. I told him things were not going well, and that we hadn't even had our first anniversary yet. I convinced him that we should get a puppy instead and that puppy would be our shared responsibility. He was thrilled with the idea, so we picked out a black Labrador retriever/Portuguese water-dog mix from our landlord's friend. Amber was great company for me on my days off and I had a ball training her. She was smart, loving, and obedient. But when Steve came home, he spoiled her rotten. He started feeding her table scraps and refused to take part in her training. The dog was getting bigger, and so was I. Steve was starting to make cracks about my extra pounds, so I geared up for a medically supervised liquid fast in the spring of 1990. Amber and I became walking partners. My body got used to the fasting pretty quickly, and as the weight melted off, my spirits started to lift and I started going out more to shop with my girlfriends. I even had the energy to go out dancing with Steve on some Friday and Saturday nights. But as the pounds dropped and I became happier and more out-going, Steve became angrier and angrier and started making irrational accusations concerning my whereabouts. Then he became so rude to my girlfriends that they began to stop calling. I was livid and felt trapped but continued to do what I wanted. He was not my father or my mother and I had to make him realize what he was doing to me and to us. Compromise was not part of my vocabulary. I was right and he was wrong, period. End of discussion. Since we only owned one car, I started asking my girlfriends to pick me up to go shopping or to lunch, but he was still angry. He wanted me to remain at home like the fat old Crystal.

One Saturday afternoon my girlfriends dropped me off around 6 P.M. after a day of shopping. Steve was already getting ready to go out for the evening. I got excited thinking about all the clothes I could finally fit into and started picking out what I wanted to wear. When he saw me all dolled up and ready to go, he told me he didn't want me to come with him. I had had my fun for the day; now it was time for him to have his fun for the night. His irrational behavior was beginning to scare me. The more I tried to reason with him, the angrier he became. That night when he arrived home, I thought I was dreaming when I looked at the clock. The club turned the lights on at 1 A.M. for the last call to order drinks. If he came straight home I would hear the key turn in the door around 1:20 A.M. When he climbed in bed that night reeking of smoke and alcohol, I thought I was going to be sick. It was 3 A.M. Sunday morning.

As my meltdown continued, he wanted to be intimate more often and started asking me to do things sexually that were way out of my comfort zone. I suspected he was doing these new kinky sexual acts with his new girlfriend. I didn't want to be touched and I certainly had no intention of accommodating his new desires. When I had to leave town on business, Steve started checking my garment bag, asking why I had to take new "sexy" underwear. When I told him I could no longer fit into my old bras and panties and to mind his own business, he started searching for other things. I was so upset I wanted to choke him. From that point on he wanted to go shopping or to lunch or to the movies with my girlfriends and me. I told him he was out of his mind and to get a life. When I'd go to the bathroom late at night, he'd ask me where I was going. I'd ignore him but if I stayed in the bathroom too long, he'd come check to see what I was doing. After weeks of arguing and angry silences he started going out all the time, not just on Friday and Saturday. When I asked him the next morning where he had been so late, he'd ignore me. The next time he left to go dancing, I waited a few hours, got dressed and went to his favorite nightspot. I sat back in the dark and watched him dance with a young lady all night. He was touching her in ways he had never touched me before and they sat close, talking intimately whenever they took a break. She had to know he was married because he was wearing his wedding ring. I wanted to go over and bust him but decided to sit back and remain cool. I wanted to take in everything he was doing so I'd have no regrets when I planned my next move. When a slow song came on, they went back to the dance floor. They danced so close together, it would have been impossible to get a razor blade between them. One of his friends had been watching me watch them and finally slithered over with a sly grin on his face and asked me to dance. I told him to wait until a fast record came on because if my husband saw me slow-dancing with his so-called buddy, someone would end up dead. Before the song ended, Steve and the young lady left. When I looked out the window he was smiling and opening the car door for her. I watched them drive off in our car around 12 A.M. I went home depressed and angry and fantasized about how I could kill him. I let Amber out to do her business and caught a glimpse of myself in the mirror. I looked fat again, but I knew that was impossible. I had just lost fifty-five pounds! I let Amber back in. I put on my nightgown and got ready for bed when the doorbell rang. I jumped and Amber started barking. I imagined there were police officers standing on the other side of the door, ready to tell me that Steve had been in a terrible car accident or had been shot. But when I looked through the peephole, it was my brother Kevin. He had a look on his face that frightened me and made me turn off the alarm and quickly unlock the door. What he told me that night changed my life—and my family's—forever.

Kevin confirmed my worst fears. He and his partner Clayton were both HIV positive. Clayton had been sick for the past few weeks and did not seem to be getting any better. Soon Kevin's and Clayton's friends were beginning to die one after the other. Kevin and I were attending funerals almost every other week, and a few weeks after that night, the last funeral we attended was Clayton's. Clayton's family threw Kevin out of Clayton's house, took all of Clayton's furniture and left town, leaving the house in shambles.

I thanked God Steve and I lived next door. Kevin came to live with us until he was able to get back on his feet, and I was thrilled. Steve, on the other hand, was initially willing to help out, but as time went on he became resentful of all the attention I gave Kevin. This was my moment to cherish every minute of time Kevin had left. I wanted to help make all of his dreams come true and pretend everything was going to be different, was going to be okay, was going to be all right.

It was one more time for me to ignore my emotions and the reality of my life. I was starting to gain back all the weight I had lost with the liquid fast. I was starting to binge again because of the stress of my marriage, which Kevin was learning about for the first time. I was also bingeing because Steve was starting to complain about Kevin living with us and nitpicked about stupid things like the way he folded towels. The weight was piling on so fast, Kevin asked what was bothering me. I just broke down and cried. I was too ashamed to tell him I felt I had no purpose in life. I hated my new job. I hated not having any friends in this new city. I hated the cost of living, I hated the crime and poverty. I hated my marriage. I hated the fact that my brother was going to die and I couldn't stop it. But most of all I hated my fat self and the way people reacted to it. I felt discriminated against in the worst way possible. Black I could handle. Female I could handle. But fat I couldn't, and I couldn't speak of that—not to Kevin, not to anybody. I didn't know where to stop or where to begin. I wanted to die.

Six months later Kevin bought his own home down the street from us. I decided to become Steve's platonic roommate and moved myself downstairs to the guest bedroom of our house. I knew Steve wasn't by himself on those nights he stayed out until the wee hours of the morning. Too many people had died already from that damned virus. I'd be a fool to let Steve touch me again. Initially, Steve was upset, but after a while he saw this as an opportunity to begin spending weekends away from home. He would pack a suitcase on Thursday, taking it with him to work that night, and would not return until Monday evening, just in time to change clothes and get ready for work that night.

One night Steve started calling around 2:30 A.M., checking up on me and wanting to make sure all the doors were locked and the alarm set. After I told him off, he stopped calling but woke me up the next morning hollering like a banshee, making crazy accusations and questioning who I had in his house the night before. He claimed there were too many dishes in the dishwasher, so I must have had someone over. I was floored and at a loss for words. Steve took that as a sign of guilt and said if he ever caught me with some n——r in his house he would shoot me and then him. The truth was there were more dishes in the dishwasher. I had started binge-ing again and had used a whole bunch of dishes for my late-night feast. Eating really was going to be the death of me. I lied and told Steve that Kevin had been over the night before, but he didn't believe me. He took off his wedding ring and announced we were no longer married.

—

Spring was Kevin's favorite time of the year because he saw it as a time of renewal and new beginnings and had prayed that his health would return. But it was the beginning of the end for him. One afternoon Kevin called me from the clinic to come for him. He had a terrible migraine and could barely see. When I arrived at the clinic, his office was dark and he was sitting with his head resting on his folded arms. The clinic was quiet. Everyone had left for the day. I gently put my arms around him and noticed, maybe not for the first time, how frail he was looking. He had lost at least thirty pounds. His shirt collar was too big around the neck and his pants were baggy and dragging on the floor. I wanted to scream and cry for mercy, but I knew I needed to remain strong for him.

When I came back to our house, Steve started in on me about where I had been. I stopped him before he went off and told him about Kevin. He calmed down and for the first time showed concern and compassion. But when I started to cry he grew nervous and began getting ready for work. He tried in his own awkward way to comfort and reassure me, but all of a sudden it was clear what a terrible, terrible mistake I had made when I settled and married out of fear. What I needed at that moment was a strong embrace from a man who loved me beyond measure. I needed to hear a confident voice reassuring me that even though things were taking a turn for the worse, God was with us and would take care of Kevin when the time came. I needed and longed to hear a man say he would be there for me and help me to take care of things when I could no longer bear another moment. Deep down I knew I was paying for the consequence of not loving myself. How could I attract someone to love and care about me if I didn't love myself first? And just to prove that I was right, that I didn't love myself, I headed to the nearest grocery store for all my favorite binge foods.

I bought four porterhouse steaks, a large bag of potato chips, four pints of Haagen-Dazs ice cream, and the makings for a peach cobbler. I stopped to check on Kevin, and when I saw how peacefully he was resting I went back home, making a mental note to mow his lawn the next day and work off my night binge. As soon as I finished preparing my feast I gave Amber a small portion of my porterhouse so she wouldn't beg for the first few minutes. I made sure I hid the rest of the food out of sight just in case Steve decided to race back home and catch me with the lover he thought I had (not a man! FOOD!) When I finished eating my first porterhouse steak with a side of potato chips, I craved something sweet. So I got my homemade peach cobbler, put a scoop of ice cream on top and watched it melt against the hot golden-brown crust. Afterward I wanted something salty again, so I ate more potato chips and a second porterhouse steak. When I got too full and felt as if I might get sick, I took an Alka-Seltzer to help break down the food. I didn't want to throw up and deal with being bulimic on top of everything else going on in my life. Then I started to cry. I cried because I was afraid I would find Kevin dead the next morning. I cried because I hated what I was doing and couldn't stop myself. I cried because I hated myself. After finally, having eaten *everything*, I felt even more miserable and took another Alka-Seltzer for relief. Before going to bed I threw away all evidence of my bingeing in time for the garbage men to pick up my secret shame. The next morning I rushed to tend to Kevin's needs, feeling headachy and bloated as if I had a hangover. My eyes, face, feet and hands were swollen. I took a deep breath before unlocking Kevin's front door. When I heard him cheerfully call out my name I thanked God for keeping him well for one more day.

I decided against telling my family how rapidly Kevin's health was deteriorating. Mom and Dad had just adopted four children, five, six, seven, and eight years old. They were all from one family and had been through years of unspeakable abuse from both their natural parents. Kelley, my younger sister, had just entered Howard University and was getting acclimated to being on her own. My brother Roy, Jr., and his wife Deborah were newlyweds and ready to start their own family. It seemed like I was the only one who could handle the truth about Kevin's health. And if it did get to be too much for me to handle, well, I would deal with that later, just like I did everything else.

Now let me tell you about those four new sisters and brothers who had just come into my life. I was really irritated at Mom for adopting those children, and for the life of me couldn't figure out why she had done it. I watched Mother struggle to raise us, particularly those summers when Dad would take off for graduate school. I watched her go back to work full-time as we grew older. I watched her go back to college. And finally I watched her come to grips with having an unplanned child nine years after I was born. My parents had thought I'd be the last one. Mom made so many sacrifices for Dad's career, moving us from state to state. She and Dad struggled to help Roy, Jr., as he became a slave to drugs, moving him in and out of rehab, finally letting go with love, and watching him recover and stand tall again. Dealing with me as a teenager and adult was no picnic either. I was fat and miserable and took it out on Mom and shut myself off from the family. And then there was Kevin. It was all my father could do to love the adult as he had loved the child and assign no guilt or blame. He did grow closer to Kevin but was filled with the grief of knowing that it would not last.

And here were these four adopted children. Mom knew Kevin was getting sicker. Why couldn't she wait to see what direction his health would take? I couldn't figure out if my parents were crazy, had too big a heart, or both. Was Mom trying to go back and re-create how she would have raised us without all the moving? Was she trying to stay busy so she wouldn't have time to think about Kevin? I didn't get it. Why did she have to make life so hard? These children were abused beyond belief by their natural parents and had been in and out of foster homes. Mom and Dad were starting all over with children who regularly referred to them as bitch and motherfucker! We would have died first before we ever fixed our mouths to say that out loud to Mom and Dad.

The phone rang and brought me back to the present. Thankfully it was my Aunt Delores. She had recently lost a significant amount of weight and I had sent her the clothes (sizes 16 to 18) that were too big for me after I had lost weight on a liquid fast. She was also asthmatic, suffered from lifelong food allergies, and had just kicked a twenty-year smoking addiction. A lot of her life had been spent in and out of hospitals. I loved my Aunt Delores and told her how proud I was of her dealing with her addictions. I also needed my clothes back! I felt bad but I couldn't afford to buy new ones. I was gaining back the weight I had lost on the liquid fast so quickly, I swore if I stood at the mirror long enough I would see the fat expanding under the layers of my skin.

A few days after Memorial Day (May 1992), I drove Kevin to Baltimore-Washington International Airport. I had called Mom and Dad ahead of time to make sure they met Kevin at the airport with a wheelchair. They still couldn't believe he was so ill and weak. When I hugged Kevin good-bye I made him promise he would return to me rested. Kevin looked at me with confidence and reassured me he was only going home for a short vacation. He made me promise that I'd take good care of his dog, Heru, especially after I took him to be neutered next week. He also asked me to keep a watchful eye on his house and car. I told him he had nothing to worry about, everything would be just fine, while my gut feeling told me this would be the last time I saw Kevin alive. When he stood up from the wheelchair to board the plane, he did not want me to help him to his seat. I watched him slowly walk away, like an old man. His left hand had developed a tremor and his skin was a shade darker than it had been, with an ashen hue. When I could no longer see his head I broke down in tears. By the time I hurried down to Kevin's car, a police officer was putting a ticket on the windshield. When I removed it to see the cost he snatched the ticket from my hand, tore it up and wrote another one for an additional twenty dollars. All I could see was the color red. When I tried to explain the situation, the officer didn't want to hear it and walked off. I wanted to take a running leap, with all my two-hundred-plus pounds, knock him to the ground and beat the living daylights out of him. But instead I let out a bloodcurdling scream. Everyone in the vicinity either stood frozen or dived to the ground for cover, with their children underneath their bodies. I drove off, crying uncontrollably, and then realized I couldn't see for my tears. I pulled over in a parking lot and watched a few planes move down the runway, all the while crying uncontrollably. After I had gained a little composure I felt exhausted and famished. I hadn't eaten all day. I drove, still crying, to the nearest Popeye's and ordered a twelve-piece Meal Deal. A moment or two later I realized I had forgotten to order something sweet, so I went back to the drive-in window. When the young girl at the window asked, with a big smirk on her face, if I had just been through there, I told her off for being ignorant, snatched my bag and told her if I came through there fifty more times she'd better not open her mouth. She uttered a nervous "Yes ma'am," and I accelerated too fast, shifting into first gear with my tires screeching loudly. Usually I would have lied or said nothing if the drive-through cashier had questioned my return so quickly. But it felt good to let out my rage!

On Friday, June 19, the phone rang and Mom said Kevin had gone home. I was numb. I couldn't believe Kevin was gone. No matter how much I had tried to prepare for the worst, I was just not prepared for his death. I can only imagine how it must feel to lose someone unexpectedly and never have the chance to say good-bye. When I told Steve, he was shocked. I called Kelley, but she wasn't home and I left a message for her to call as soon as possible. I put a leash on Heru and we walked down to Kevin's house and went to his third-floor bedroom. I walked outside onto his deck with its partial view of downtown and I looked toward the harbor, where we had watched fireworks on the Fourth of July and New Year's Eve. I was looking for a sign from Kevin telling me that he was all right. We had always promised one another that if anything happened, if one of us did go to the other side, and if we made it "safely," we would send a signal of flashing lights. And that is what I was waiting for—those flashing lights. After about twenty minutes I started crying and sat down with Heru by my side, just praying that Kevin was at peace. When I turned around to look down into the yard, there was a bright light shining. Kevin's floodlights, which had not worked since the day he moved into the house, were on!

My tears of sorrow turned to tears of joy as I jumped up and down looking at the floodlights. Heru jumped around the deck with me as I yelled, "Everything's gonna be all right, everything's gonna be all right!" Steve showed up about then to say that Kelley had called and I needed to call her back. When I showed him the floodlights were on, he couldn't believe it. After Steve had left, I stood there a little longer with Heru, not wanting to let go of my last moment with Kevin. This was the way I wanted to remember his spirit, flooding the night with brightness. I turned my head for a split second to catch a sound inside the house and when I turned around again, it was pitch-black.

—

June 19 is known in African-American history as Juneteenth, the day our ancestors were freed from slavery in 1865. June 19 is also my Uncle Andrew's birthday and the birth date and death date of my great-grandmother. It was the day Steve and I closed on our first home, and finally, it was the day Dad was supposed to fly back to Baltimore with Kevin. No one, not even me, could predict there was more turmoil to come.

From August 1992–September 1993 one horrible event after another happened.

In August, Hurricane Andrew destroyed my parents' home in Florida. In December, 1992, I had a partial hysterectomy and Steve announced he would now have to have children outside of marriage. In April, 1993, my beloved Aunt Delores died a few days after coming home from the hospital. And in September, 1993, I finally left Steve. The next fifteen months were filled with despair, with long nights of bingeing, with hopeless self-loathing. I went in search of peace and found only despair. The scale climbed steadily and finally came to rest just under the three-hundred-pound mark. Desperate to move quickly away from three hundred pounds, I started taking diet pills and starved off forty-seven pounds, putting me at two hundred forty-five pounds. I knew I couldn't continue losing weight this way and gave up the diet pills. The pounds started to pile on again and my old eating patterns were in full swing. I was sick to death of being on a diet; I felt horrible in everything I put on; I was increasingly depressed. I knew the girlfriends I had in my life were my friends only because I made them look good and I was no threat to them, especially when we went out to parties. So I started turning down their invites to go out and distanced myself from them. I lived by watching the world through TV or by talking on the phone.

New Year's Eve 1994 was the turning point. One of my girlfriends called me and asked me to go to a New Year's Eve service with her and her boyfriend. I only went because I had been promising her that I'd visit her church and thought this would keep her quiet for a while.

I don't remember much about that New Year's Eve sermon now, but whatever it was, it made me go home and take a long look at myself. I surrendered to God's power and love and confessed that I had too much of *other* people's baggage in my life and was neglecting my own. My life force was running on empty, and the only way to rejuvenate it was to rejuvenate me. I decided to watch an old "Oprah Winfrey" tape. In this particular episode, Oprah talked about her second dramatic weight loss and challenged her viewing audience to embark on a journey of self-discovery by journal writing and reexamining the painful periods of their lives. Not by eating, not by bingeing, but by feeling the feelings and letting them go. I hadn't been ready for this message the first time I'd heard it and I wasn't sure I was ready for it now. I just didn't believe I was holding on to things that had happened so long ago. Hadn't I resolved all of that? I didn't want to feel any more pain and feared what might come if I reopened the past. I was comfortable believing food was my problem. Was I ready? Was I at my wit's end? Could I continue to live the rest of my life feeling purposeless? What about that "one more time" promise I had made to God just a few weeks ago? Hadn't I learned from Kevin and Aunt Delores that life was too short? Hadn't I learned that pleasing and loving should always start with myself first? I wanted a chance to get it right.

I admired Oprah for all the hard work she put into losing weight. I admired her for doing it the right way, for never giving up and never being afraid to try again in the face of those who would love to see her fail again. But how could I do it? How could I achieve my goal? I was still only working part-time, I wasn't rich, and I didn't have my own personal trainer. My family lived several states away and I was still grieving over the loss of my brother and aunt. Therapy wasn't an option at the moment. I didn't have the money, and the therapist I did see toward the end of my marriage had struck just a little too close to home. Oprah had said something about a journal, and that seemed as good as anything. In time my journal would become my safe haven, the therapist's couch, best friend, and a sanctuary all rolled into one. But now it was just a place to start. Somehow I knew I was ready to confront the demons in my life. I was ready to put my emotional road map on paper. I was ready to do the work.

Thank you, Oprah.

4

A CHANGE IS GONNA COME

December 31, 1994

> Here I am at 245 lbs. trying to get down to 133 lbs. Am I
> fooling myself, or what? I feel HUGE! I visited a friend's
> church to bring in the New Year and asked God to help me
> get down to the fabulous weight I know I can achieve. I
> didn't feel like going up to the altar to pray, fearing I
> wouldn't be able to get back up, so I prayed in the safety of
> the pews. I shouldn't have worn this skirt (size 22). It's cut-
> ting me in half.

After my story appeared in *Essence, Fitness, Ebony* and *Living Fit* magazines and especially after I appeared on "The Remembering, Spirit" segment of the "Oprah Winfrey show," people from all over the world contacted me. The number-one question everyone always asks is "How did you stay motivated over the long haul, and what keeps you motivated now?" My response is always. "I stopped dieting." That's the easy answer. The harder answer is I had to find out what all the extra weight was really saying to me about me. That meant I had to stop dieting, to stop worrying about food, so I could work on some other things first.

What amazes me after all the years of thinking I was a failure because I could never stick to a diet is that food was never the problem! It was just a *symptom* of the problem(s). For years I was in denial about what was really eating away at me. Isn't that ironic? I was eating because something was eating me. I was reluctant to do the work or face anything that smacked of being honest about my feelings. I didn't want to go back to my childhood and reexperience the pain of feeling ugly and worthless. Or deal with the reason I had started bingeing. I didn't want to admit that my mental development was as arrested as my lust for life.

The bottom line? Deciding to face my past saved my life. No one but me could work through the years of accumulated fear, anger, guilt, and unworthiness. It took time and it took courage, but I was determined not to be a failure statistic. I had a lot of work to do, and my journal is one of the places where I started. I needed to write about the fear and anger, guilt and worthlessness to understand why I loved food more than I loved myself. I'll talk more about my journal later, because as you'll see, my journal was a place for me to clean house.

I realize not everyone who is overweight or obese binges. I realize not everyone who needs to lose weight is eating because of past childhood traumas. But for the people who are ready to admit they are using food to silence pain, I'd like to share with you the steps I took to heal and free myself of the excess baggage. After I lost weight so many people came to me asking for help that I decided to start my own weight-loss workshops locally and soon began traveling to speak to groups across the country.

So for those of you who never had an opportunity to hear how I changed myself from the inside out, roll up your sleeves and prepare to do some heavy-duty housecleaning. In the words of Sam Cooke's song, "A change is gonna come!"

Find the Root of the Problem

Let's face it, reflecting on the past and dealing with it is painful, and that's why most people fight changing what is right in front of them. It is much easier just to continue on the same way, investing in food, sex, alcohol, drugs, gossip, endless hours in front of the TV or computer—anything to escape, anything to avoid change or action. Think of it as pulling the roots of a dandelion out of your lawn—you have to go to the root of your unhappiness to get rid of it.

When I finally put pen to pad and started writing about my day and my relationship with food and people, I began to see eating patterns. I saw that bingeing provided me with an emotional release in situations I felt I couldn't handle. Binges stopped my emotional and spiritual growth, so I was stuck emotionally at eight years old because that's when I stopped dealing with life.

Binges were my misguided way of giving something back to myself. Food seemed to give me everything I felt had been taken from me as an obese African-American woman. When I binged I became a victim. I was tired of the experts telling me that to be beautiful I had to be a certain race, or, almost as bad, a certain shade of skin color, weight, height, or age. Food was legal, cheap, readily available twenty-four hours a day, and I never had to worry about being pulled over while driving under the influence of a food binge. Food made me feel complete, especially carbohydrates and sweets. The minute I had one or the other I was lifted into a euphoric state. But hours later I'd come crashing down, more depressed than ever, and start the vicious cycle of punishing myself for not being able to stick to another diet. While it lasted, it felt great . . .

In 1993, before I left Steve, I made one last desperate attempt to hold on to my doomed marriage. In retrospect, I see that the sessions I had with a local therapist, Audrey Chapman, helped me tremendously, but at the time they felt mean and painful. Even though I wasn't eager to air my dirty laundry with a stranger, I had convinced Steve to go with me. I had listened to Audrey's talk show on WHUR radio out of Washington, D.C. and respected her work. But when she finished with me, I was steaming.

First, I resented that she only had two sessions with Steve and me before suggesting I come for counseling by *myself.* Secondly, Audrey read me like a book, from day one, and knew I was full of you-know-what. After I told her about my childhood and my relationship with other men, she told me exactly why I was attracted to my husband. Steve and I were the perfect match for one another because we kept the drama going. Bingeing and dieting created the perfect stage for my drama and Steve fed right into it. Compulsive eating represented everything I loved about theater and daytime soap operas: hope, fear, excitement, passion, anticipation, happiness, rage, grief, sorrow, and illusion. No wonder I had sizes 9 through 24 in my closet. That drama didn't start with my marriage, though. I had a long history of theater.

The summers my father was away at graduate school, I would feel sorry for Mom, and to forget *her* pain I would sneak into the kitchen, stuff Ritz crackers into my underwear and eat them in the backyard under the cherry tree. I would fantasize about Dad coming home and throwing Mom into a dip—holding her steady in his arms while she kicked one leg into the air and laughed at the wonderful silliness of it all. Then they would kiss and be full of passion to make up for all the lonely times.

When Dad did come home they did embrace and kiss, but I wanted more—something more like in the movies or the soaps. Within a few days the thrill would be gone between Mom and Dad. Dad would drop back into his routine of going downstairs to his study or prepare for work. Mom would get mad because he would ignore us for days on end. Then the arguments would start. Mom would usually storm up to their bedroom crying and Dad would follow. I would hear them talking for hours and then silence. Dad would go to the store and always bring back Mom's favorites for dinner and then we'd all eat together. If the Good Humor ice cream truck came around and Mom wanted dessert, that meant dessert for everyone! I soon learned that behavior and love and emotions were all connected with food.

Audrey told me that I chose men who were not available to me emotionally. When I met Steve, he gave me everything I thought I wanted emotionally, but when it was more than enough, it began to suffocate me. I pulled back, demanding space, and he went into jealous rages. My fears kept me from looking inside myself for answers. I was too busy playing victim and pointing to others for my misfortunes. Audrey told me that being a victim was not my fault, but staying one was, and as an adult, I was responsible for what I did with my pain. I was ready to put in earplugs right about then.

In my last session with Audrey, she rhetorically and gently threw out some questions that made me think. The answers made me finally leave my husband. "What do you think living with someone like your husband for the rest of your life will do to your health? He is not equipped to change and has told you he isn't going to change." I hated her because I knew she was right. Yet even though my husband was to blame as well as me, she respected his honesty. I saw him as a stubborn ol' goat! I hated her because even though her intention was not to embarrass or humiliate me, that was how I felt.

"Why do you choose to live your life like this when you are capable of change? Why are you wasting your life? Why are you unwilling to end this wall of silence with your parents?"

And finally I hated her because she saw how manipulative I was. Wasn't I the one looking for sympathy and pity during our first visit, pouring out my sob story about my partial hysterectomy?

Audrey never told me what to do, but she gave me tons to think about. I was still acting out my childhood, trying to please my father by getting better grades in math and science. I was as silent in my marriage as I had been in class when my first- and second-grade teachers laughed at me when I gave wrong answers. I still resented my mother for not protecting me from my grandfather. I was so wrapped up in my past that there was no way I could live in the present.

As soon as I opened myself up for change, became angry, grieved, forgave and let it go, the weight started disappearing. It's not easy going into the medicine cabinet of your mind, but it beats everything else I've tried. I'm still a work in progress, but with time and more healing, it's getting easier. Remember that until you release the pain, you will continue to gain weight. Think about what the extra weight represents to you. Is it saying I can't, I hurt, I'm sad, come closer, go away, leave me alone, love me? Do you even know what or when you eat, or is it just a reflex? You may not be able to get to the root of why you eat compulsively right away. This process may be gradual and come to you in stages.

Here are a few more of my early journal entries and my first steps towards healing.

January 3, 1995

> Last night I had a dream that disturbed me all day today. All I can remember was that I was trapped in a room that I could not get out of for hours. When someone finally opened the door to let me out, it was Grandfather. I was upset over this all day and started eating over it. I'm afraid to go to sleep tonight because I'm afraid what my dream will reveal.

January 4, 1995

When the alarm went off this morning I shut it off and rolled back over. I knew it was cold out today because the heat stayed on for most of the night. The alarm went off again after another ten minutes, but I stayed in bed. Heru (my dog) pawed the mattress continuously. He was anxious to go outside to do his business. I finally got up and let him out. The cold air woke me up so I decided to exercise before going to work. The journey of a thousand miles begins with a single step.

January 5, 1995

Had a dream about Kevin last night. I dreamed we were living in Detroit again, standing on Seven Mile waiting for the bus to take us to Cass Tech High School. Our bus never came, so we walked to school and had a long discussion about what I needed to do to lose weight this time. Kevin told me to start dealing with my fears so I would be able to respect myself again. I was shocked because I didn't realize my fears were so transparent. Before the dream ended he told me to stop living my life in fear.

Building a Strong Foundation for Your Motivation

My motivation to lose weight had to be more than wanting to wear that size 8 for the next wedding or reunion, because what would be my motivation when that event was over? Proving I had will power and wanting to look good to men wouldn't be enough. My motivation had to come from deep down inside. It had to be about the way I felt when I went to bed and got up again the next morning. I had to love the face in the mirror because I was worth it. What I needed more than anything was to love myself enough to want to live and be healthy.

Let Go and Let God

Holding on to hate was killing me inside. Holding on to past
regrets and guilt made me weak. Seeking revenge and plotting it
out in my dreams was driving me mad. I had to stop judging all
fair-skinned African-Americans. I had to stop seeing discrimination in every white face and place. I had to come to terms with not
being able to control or change what others thought about me. I
had a full-time job in just working on me. I would let God take
care of everything else.

January 10, 1995

> I can't believe I'm up at 2 A.M. writing, but I'm so angry I
> can't sleep. First, I have to thank God for Charlotte, my dis-
> trict manager and mentor. If it had not been for her, and my
> best friend Katrina, I would not have landed this job (six
> years ago) with a major pharmaceutical company on their
> flex-time sales force. I had been interviewing for a year with
> other pharmaceutical companies but never made it past the
> final interview—usually with a regional manager. Despite
> having five years of previous successful sales experience, I
> always got the thumbs-down. And then someone finally told
> me the truth—I was too fat! My goal has always been to prove
> myself and move to the full-time sales force selling prescrip-
> tion medications instead of over-the-counter medications.
> Charlotte told me today that a full-time position has opened
> up right here in the Baltimore area, but when I asked her if it
> would be offered to me she hesitated and said to be patient,
> which I knew meant her boss didn't want to give me the posi-
> tion. A reliable source in home office told me he was doing
> everything in his power to block me from getting this full-
> time position. I'm going to get it anyway but this s.o.b. is
> going to make my life miserable. My inside home office

source also said they would fill this position tomorrow and legally they have to give it to me. I was so upset I couldn't eat all day after hearing the news.

But now I could eat a house! I know I shouldn't eat now, but dammit, I'm really hungry. Okay, take a deep breath. Why not try a cup of herbal tea with honey and an orange? Anyway, back to this miserable man. I've always noticed, whenever I'm around him, he watches me like a hawk—just waiting for me to mess up—but I've never let him see me sweat. After I left my husband, my hair was so badly damaged from perms and stress that I cut it all off and now I'm sporting a short natural Caesar cut. When he saw me at one of our national sales meetings he made a negative comment and then quickly recovered and started showering me with compliments each time he saw me. He made sure he said this in the company of his golf companions. Hair is very political for African-American women. My experience is that if our hair is not straightened with a relaxer, then insecure people think you're militant and become very threatened. I've even noticed some of the doctors I do business with looking at me differently and acting uneasy. I struggled with the decision of going natural just because of this stupidity. I even had a brother complain in my presence that he wished women would stop trying to go for that "Toni Braxton" look because the women are starting to look like lesbians. I wanted to drop-kick his butt but stuffed my mouth with food instead at the party. All I wanted was a healthy head of hair and simplicity when I exercised. Amazing what one little head can do . . . Most of all I'm angry because I have allowed this horrid man to steal my joy. Tomorrow he will be the one to offer me the full-time position and the added responsibility of being the district trainer. I have managed to get through my brother's death, Aunt Delores's death, my hysterectomy, the struggle to leave my husband, and Hurricane Andrew's destruction of my parent's home. I am stronger than he is. I will do the right thing. I will be the bigger person.

Arthur Ashe was so right when he questioned how much time and energy was taken up in his life dealing with racism. Not only do I have to deal with the color thing, but I also have to deal with being a woman and being overweight. I will come out on top—it is just going to take some time, some crying, a lot of healing and prayer and recommitting every day to a new way of living.

Eliminate or Spend Less Time Around Negative People

It takes a lot of energy to be positive, but it takes no effort to be negative. After shedding most of my excess baggage, I was surprised at the number of people I encountered who thrived on negativity. Just like animals can spot weak ones in a pack when targeting to attack, so can miserable people.

These people are not your friends. Get rid of them. You have nothing to lose and you'll gain back your self-respect in the process. As for family members, well, there's always a rotten one in the barrel, isn't there? Be cordial, be polite, and leave it at that. We inherit our family, we choose our friends. If you happen to live with a family member who would qualify for the negative sign on the end of your battery, God bless you. Get help if you can. Single ladies learn to look for the red flags and early warning signs in relationships. Dump losers early and move on. Reexamine your expectations for this person and the relationship. And just keep on doing your own work.

January 12, 1995

Still thinking about that dream I had a few weeks ago. I've decided that I will get rid of all the people in my life that are negative. Last week I had a falling-out with two girlfriends over some he-said-she-said mess. Both only had me around to make themselves look better. They could not stand one another and one of them said I was not being a good friend by being friends with someone she did not like. Thank goodness they are no longer in my life. From now on I will not let just anyone enter my life. All my life I've let people talk to me and treat me like an old rag doll. This will be the beginning of my healing process. I will only allow a loving and nurturing environment around me and people who are supportive and positive. If I'm going to start loving myself I have to demand that others respect me as well. Being malleable is a trait that no longer suits my life.

Eliminate Negative Self-talk
Lord knows there're enough negative people walking around who can't wait to rain on your parade. So start being kind to yourself and challenge yourself to change your inner voice. I had to retrain my inner voice to speak positively about me. Instead of thinking, "I can't fit my big behind into that outfit," I'd stop and correct my inner voice by saying, "One day soon, I *will* be able to fit into that outfit. I will feel good and look fabulous in it, too!" When you continue to think and talk negatively you produce negative behavior and limit yourself. You also invite other negative people to take digs at you. When you begin treating yourself with kindness, others around you will follow suit and you'll attract positive people into your life.

Being kind to yourself also helps you to forgive yourself. Don't forget that changing your behavior is a process and you may still be in the mode of beating yourself up when you fail. Remember not to fall into that trap. If you've eaten too much, don't say or think, "Well I've blown it and may as well eat the rest and start again first thing tomorrow," or "I can't even get through two hours without blowing it; forget this, I'm just meant to be fat." Don't go there! We're babies learning how to walk again. Get up, brush yourself off, and start learning from that incident. Discover what made you eat nonstop. Taking time to learn from that eating episode will take you to a higher level of learning about what triggers your eating and about yourself. It will also give you clues about your needs and motivations and help you the next time it happens. And there will be a next time. Trust me, I know. Hopefully, if you're seeking permanent change, you'll find the more you practice this remedial thinking, the quicker you'll be able to catch a lapse and not allow it to go into a relapse. Best of all, write it down.

January 16, 1995

> Today was not a good day for me. I wasn't satisfied with anything I ate all day, so I started eating all my old junk food that ended up making me sick. I didn't exercise because I felt so bad about what I ate and had no energy. I know I can't have another day like this one. This is how my diets usually end and I end up gaining back all the weight I had lost. This time I will NOT give up on me again. I'm gonna make me love me!—"Change—A bend in the road is not the end of the road unless you fail to make the turn."—Corporate Impressions, Successories, Lombard, Illinois

I mentioned *trigger* foods. Do you know about trigger foods? Trigger foods are usually salty or sweet and it is almost impossible to eat just one or two spoonfuls—like peanuts or potato chips or M&Ms or ice cream; the list goes on and on. Trigger foods are often the first thing you think about when you are angry or depressed or upset. They aren't so bad in themselves, but the first bite is like the top of a sliding board: once you start down, you just keep going and going and going. Pay attention to what you grab for if you are having a bad day. Write it down and see if it happens more than once or twice. Is there a pattern?

Sit Down with Family and Friends and Ask for Their Help

Donna Britt of the *Washington Post* asked in a column, "How often do Black women ask for what we need?" Ladies, as a compulsive eater I was also a compulsive giver. I knew how to nurture, help, and listen to others. Since I would not allow myself to accept the same in return, I continued the vicious cycle of pleasing others and leaving myself empty. I had problems setting limits and did not know how to say no because I wanted to feel loved and respected by others. Those on the receiving end soon start to expect this from you and will run you till you drop.

So begin retraining yourself and learn to fix your mouth around NO! When you are tired, ask for help. Get out of that Aunt Jemima syndrome. Taking care of yourself takes practice—especially if you have never felt worthy. Grow a second layer of skin, become tough, and be prepared for others to make you feel guilty for starting to care more for yourself. When they start to call you selfish or say that you have changed, *don't* let that guilt-trip you back into that Aunt Jemima mode! Remember, nurturing yourself is the key. It's like filling your car up with gas when it's on empty. Just as a car will stop without fuel, your body will, too. I've seen many of my relatives leave before their time because they didn't stop to take their asthma medication, or they felt better so they stopped taking their hypertension medication, or they did not refill medications—hoping to save money to provide more for the family.

Now is the time to sit down with family and friends to discuss what changes you want to make in your life and what kind of support you need from them. Whatever you do, *please* don't tell them that you're going on another diet because you're not. You're making a permanent lifestyle change. Your friends and family can share in your new healthy awareness of food, not in tasteless, limited choices. This is the time to break the vicious cycle of passing down bad eating habits from generation to generation. This is a wonderful time to help your children change their eating habits.

Do not allow or assign anyone to be your food police. You have to be responsible for your own self-development. *Now, go on and set the tone for yourself and your family.*

Accept Your Reality Now

Accepting the way you look today doesn't mean that you shouldn't work toward a better tomorrow. If you were in a burning house and standing next to an open door, would you run out to save yourself? I sure hope so! Well, now is the time to start saving yourself and believing in yourself again. Accept that you weigh too much today, set no time frame, and start building your new brick house for a better tomorrow.

Initially, it was difficult for me to accept that I had over a hundred and fifty pounds to lose. But I knew if I continued to think about the negative, I'd never move forward. It's difficult to hope again, especially if you've been overweight all your life. But let's take a moment and look at things a little differently. God has given *you* all the tools and resources on this earth to be healthy. He gave you a mind so powerful, you only use a fraction of it in your daily life. Use what God has given you this time. Don't starve yourself, don't rush the process. Find a way to enjoy the process of your metamorphosis. Pick an old photograph of yourself. Choose and visualize a goal that is attainable. Let *no one* tell you that your goal is unattainable.

Now I'm going to ask you to do something that may be very uncomfortable. Stand in front of a full-length mirror totally nude. Then move closer to the mirror and stare at your face and say, "I love you." I was horrified that I could not do something so simple. I cried when I said "I love you." It was tough, but I forced myself to stand there and repeat it over and over and over again. You will not begin to move forward until you can embrace yourself, alone, with your face and body in the mirror.

Please don't just read this and move on. DO IT! It is truly powerful and will be one of the building blocks of your recovery. Next, force yourself to stand in front of a full-length mirror every day and pick ONE thing you like about your body and ONE thing you want to improve. It was tough for me to pick even one thing when I weighed more than two hundred pounds, so I started with my teeth and went from there. It took me forever to stop myself from pointing out everything I wanted to improve. It was tough for me to use kind, gentle words and not harsh, degrading ones when I finally pinpointed a spot for fine-tuning. Even though I felt just the opposite, I performed this ritual on a daily basis. At first I felt stupid and uncomfortable. But with time, effort and practice, it became easier and easier—and *I started to believe what I was saying.*

January 17, 1995

Kuji, Kevin's best friend, suggested I develop a mantra. She said the mantra should contain positive affirmations to reinforce the way I want to feel about myself. So this morning I looked in the mirror and stared at my reflection for a long, long time. Then I hugged myself and told myself that I loved me. I also started telling myself what I loved most about me physically. I loved my even-toned skin, full lips and nose. I loved my almond-shaped eyes. I felt silly and uncomfortable, but I promised myself I would perform this ritual every morning until I believed every word I said. I love my hair now that it is healthy and natural, but I'm starting to grow tired of my short natural Caesar haircut. I want a more feminine look, something that will make me look softer and allow me to create a different hairstyle on different days. My sister Kelley encouraged me to do something that would promote hair growth and be almost maintenance-free—braids. Glorious braids!

Set No Time Limit on Your Weight Loss

When a new member of my weight-loss workshop asks, "How long do you think it will take me to lose fifty pounds?" I know she is only looking for a temporary change. My ladies look at me as if I'm crazy when I say, "Is there a way for children to skip the crawling phase before they start walking? Can they just skip crawling and advance on to walking automatically?" Just as there are no short-cuts to a child's development, there are no shortcuts to losing weight quickly and keeping it off permanently. Weight loss happens slowly, without force, and takes time and patience.

There were days when I felt like giving up and had to find a way to recommit. I'd play mind games with myself when I craved my old binge foods. I would say, "Okay, Crystal, you can go to Popeye's for your twelve-piece meal deal and make some homemade peach cobbler, but wait fifteen more minutes to go out, and do your paperwork first." I'd keep playing the game until I forgot about what it was I wanted or went to bed mad because trying to retrain that spoiled child was hard work. I really did want to change, so I had to stop myself at age thirty-four and reach back for the eight-year-old I left behind in 1968. I had to find out why she was mad and why she was trying to heal herself with not just one piece of fried chicken but *ten pieces!*

Committing to change means reprogramming your mind and getting rid of fad diets and quick-weight-loss schemes that work about as well as get-rich-quick schemes. How many times has the weight you lost found you again? If you can't continue to eat the way you are eating (to lose weight), then you are on a diet. STOP! Stop dieting, start eating, and trust the process. *You are not alone and you will be successful.*

These are all the things that helped me, motivated me and moved me forward. I am not a trained counselor or psychologist, but what I have learned and put into practice comes from the heart and years of practical experience. When other women come to me and ask for help, this is where we start. You will read some of their stories later.

Ask yourself why you bought this book. Did you really want to read about my story, or did you think that maybe I was going to offer a magic solution? Sorry, but my weight loss was work.

5

LOOKING GOOD
TO YOU OR TO HIM?

*O*kay ladies, it's time for a very touchy subject. I want you to know that I speak from *my* experience in *my* workshops. My work as a motivational speaker has given me valuable insight about why we, as African-Americans, often suffer with our weight.

Culturally, full-figured women are celebrated in traditional African societies, and many of us, men and women, have embraced this as a standard of beauty today. Being large is also equated with "living large" or living well—and who among us does not want to be thought of as successful? The problem is that this heritage is based on a life where drought, famine, even death, were commonplace. When is the last time you went without food or water for days, or with very little food for weeks, perhaps even months? When is the last time you were forcibly moved from your homeland? There is great nostalgia and longing for us to be connected with the lands of our ancestors, but we, no matter what we think, do not live as they did and as some Africans still do.

Instead, we live in a land of fast cars, fast-food restaurants, artificial sweeteners, and calorie-laden but fat-free cookies. Our ancestors walked more in one day than most of us do in a month. They ate fruits and vegetables, nuts and berries. They ate only what they grew or killed. Yes, we have a wonderful and notable heritage, but let us understand it within the context of our life today.

A few years ago I flew to California for my grandmother's funeral, knowing I would see relatives I had not seen in years. I dreaded going and almost didn't go because I was at my all-time high of 292 pounds. I prayed my relatives would have the grace not to mention my weight but I knew that was just wishful thinking. When the plane landed I said another silent prayer, hoping one particular loudmouth uncle would not be standing there at the gate with my father. I could just hear it now, "My God! I know that ain't Crystal! Girl, you're as big as a house!" *Mind you, I do own a mirror. I do look in it occasionally and I do know I'm dragging around another person. Hello! I am aware of what I look like, thank you very much!*

Thank goodness that uncle wasn't there, but another one saw me and from him I got, "Whoa! I didn't recognize you, baby. You're so big!" I had been bracing for just this welcome and replied with a very stoic, "Hello, and how are you?" When he sensed my shame, discomfort, and wind chill, he responded immediately, "But, baby, all that means is that you're living well." Now that comment may have worked if my tribe of immediate family members had just escaped a drought or were recovering from a famine, but, trust me, that wasn't the case.

In the early eighties I often called on doctors whose offices were in poor sections of Baltimore and the conversations I heard in those waiting rooms were enough to make chills run up my back: Once I overheard a woman explaining to her girlfriend that she was glad she was fat because then men would know she wasn't dying of AIDS or hooked on crack. I was floored but started to understand why some of my sisters felt comfortable and even flaunted being overweight. What a sad commentary on our society that we use fat to say what we are not instead of what we are. That being fat is the opposite of being sick.

Surveys in this country show that most white women are dissatisfied with their bodies, but African-American women are not. Typically, African-American women are satisfied with their body type, no matter what the size, while even the slimmest of white women voice concern about their size. Clinical psychologist Jeanette Harris noticed the attitude difference years ago in college students and started studying how African-American women and Caucasian women viewed their bodies. She says, "Television tells us what Caucasian women should look like: thin equals attractiveness. Caucasian women have often been seen as the standard of beauty, and that's too great a standard to have to live up to." That fits perfectly with what Susan Taylor, publication director of *Essence* magazine, says. Ms. Taylor noted that African-American men and women, because of long-held white stereotypes in the fashion industry, have not, until recently, had visual images of what they could look like, so they created their own image. We created an image that complimented our body type and heritage.

The attitude difference is even more dramatic in teenage girls. One study shows that seventy percent of African-American girls reported being happy with their bodies, versus only ten percent of Caucasian girls. Dr. Harris suggests this might be due to the narrow view of attractiveness Caucasians have set for themselves, while in the African-American community "there is a greater range of what we call attractive and beautiful, even if we are significantly overweight." Ms. Taylor goes on to say that because our beauty has been defiled for hundreds of years, it has taught us to close our ears to what other people might have to say about our bodies (and hair). (Information from *20/20* TV segment.)

Let's go back even further and examine a report about African women and their view of their bodies after immigration from Africa to Great Britain. A study by Furnham and Alibhai (1983)—

(Studies from "The Body Betrayed—A deeper Understanding of Women, Eating Disorders, and Treatment," by Kathryn, J. Zerbe, M.D.) notes that fatness has traditionally been a greater preoccupation of Western society than Third World countries. African women were generally comfortable with fuller figures and embraced their size with brightly colored robes and headdresses. But, just four years after relocating to Great Britain, those same women adopted the British viewpoint with respect to size and shape, as compared to their African peers. The report went on to say that the British women favored an almost anorexic body size. These Kenyan women were also, in the course of those four years, eating very differently. The context of their heritage had changed.

We have to go beyond what we know culturally and perhaps what our men want physically, and rightly start placing value in ourselves and in our *health*. Am I glad that we, as African-American women, can be happy with our different body sizes? Absolutely. Remember, I'm not talking skinny. I'm not talking about being a model wanna-be, I'm not even talking about being a certain size, I am talking healthy. Substituting hypertension and diabetes drugs for nutrition and exercise is not healthy. Eating when your are not physically hungry is not healthy. Carrying thirty or fifty extra pounds just because your man likes a big behind is not healthy. Not exercising and not eating fruits and vegetables is not healthy. It's really very simple. Fat is killing African-American mothers, wives, sisters, and daughters. Fat is killing us and we are passing on our obesity from generation to generation.

The National Institute of Health reports "Every year obesity-related conditions account for three hundred thousand deaths in the United States and are regarded as the second leading preventable cause of death after smoking." Further, "fifteen years ago the average woman wore a size 12. Today the average woman wears a size 14."

The National Center on Addiction and Substance Abuse says

"Women over 59 years of age take an average of five prescriptions at the same time."

And just in case you think I am alone in this cause, think again. Look at what has happened as African-Americans move into the spotlight—whether in government, business, music, theater, television, advertising, movies, or a myriad other areas. Our bodies become a representation of ourselves and how we relate to the world. Think about Angela Bassett, Jennifer Holiday, Janet Jackson, Patti LaBelle, and, of course, Oprah Winfrey. I've noticed from listening and talking with members of my weight-loss workshops that just as we want a fine-looking man, our brothers are moving toward an appreciation of a more streamlined and healthy body. Think about it this way: Have you ever seen Will Smith or Denzel Washington or Babyface or Magic Johnson or Michael Jordan with a less than well-toned woman on his arm? Remember, I'm not talking skinny, I'm talking healthy.

I know that getting healthy—mentally, physically and spiritually—is no easy feat. But we are survivors! Despite genocide, despite slavery, despite years of segregation and discrimination, we are still here. Surely we can find the strength and courage to tap into that spirit of survival and use it to be our best selves. This is not a call to follow the image of what some would have us believe is ideal, but it is a call to live to our full potential, to live in health, and to live in such a way that we can nourish and be nourished by more than just food. I want you to know that extraordinary feeling of looking in the mirror and saying to the beautiful, healthy image staring back—I LOVE YOU!

After losing my 157 pounds I remember going to meet some friends at the Rusty Scupper in Baltimore's Inner Harbor. The sun was starting to set and it was a beautiful evening—a perfect time to take a stroll with that special someone. I was feeling good about my accomplishments and slowed my pace, remembering the summers I spent with my ex-husband walking this same territory as an unhappy, obese woman. If I saw an attractive, fit woman approaching us, I'd become insecure and ask what he thought of her. He'd respond with, "She's too thin." And I would feel better until I'd catch a glimpse of myself in a shop window. That evening as I approached an African-American couple (she was heavy and he was average weight) who were sitting on a bench, I overheard her asking him what he thought of me. His response was. "She's too thin." I smiled and slowed my pace as I then approached a Caucasian couple who were both an average weight. I was floored when I heard her asking him what he thought about me. When he said I was a little too heavy, I almost burst into laughter because it confirmed what I had known for a while. I was j-u-s-t right!

6

BUILDING BLOCKS:
WHAT TO EAT

*L*ike every overweight woman I know, I was an expert on calorie counts, fat-grams counts, protein counts, and carbohydrate counts. You name it, I knew it. But what I didn't know was what would work for me over the long haul. What you have to find, just like I did, are your building blocks, or food bricks, and lay the foundation for a day of feeling good and feeling satisfied. And just like building a house, it's a matter of putting one brick on top of another.

Let me tell you first what did not work for me. In the year and a half before I knelt in that church pew and asked God to help me change my life, I had starved off forty-seven pounds with the help of a very popular prescription drug. The weight melted off because I didn't eat—a banana or tuna-fish sandwich might be it for an entire day. In the meantime, I was bouncing off the walls with the highest of highs and the lowest of lows. I'm supposed to be a smart lady, a college graduate, and here I was, working for a pharmaceutical company that did random drug testing (if you were suspect), and on a good day I was flying about three feet above the sidewalk. I wasn't eating, I wasn't sleeping, and I was exercising on chemical energy. Finally, terrified of losing my job, and exhausted from the daily battle my body was waging, I asked my doctor to wean me off the drugs. Six weeks later, as I approached that fateful New Year's Eve, all my old eating patterns were beginning to surface and I was starting to gain weight. Something, everything had to change.

January 18, 1995

> I'm sick of checking fat grams and I'm sick of feeling deprived! I know I shouldn't give up now, but just thinking about how much weight I have to lose discourages me. There's no light at the end of this tunnel. I've got to find a way to keep going because I'm running out of willpower. I'm having dreams of peach cobbler, but I know if I start eating that way again I may as well be dead.

My usual dieting cycle went something like this:

> Start rabbit-food diet on Monday.
> Rapid weight loss (usually water).
> Weight loss slows down until scale shows no change.
> Get frustrated and pissed off.
> Drive to the nearest Popeye's Chicken with an attitude and binge.
> Vow to exercise to work off the twelve-piece meal deal.
> Fall asleep instead on the living room sofa with the TV and exercise bike watching me.
> Beat myself up for failing again and wonder if I'll ever lose weight.
> Vow to start fresh again on Monday.

I was eating no-fat everything and wasn't satisfied by any of it, mentally or physically. I was using a lot of frozen and canned low-fat products, and after eating a "fat-controlled, portion-controlled" meal I was generally left with an empty feeling. I was irritable, particularly after dinner, and would find myself tapping my foot nervously. And then, before the evening was over, I would be rummaging through the cabinets and refrigerator like a raccoon until I found something that *satisfied* me.

January 20, 1995

> Horrible food day. Ate continuously all day long even though I wasn't hungry. I knew I was eating too much but I just couldn't stop. I sat around all evening, watching TV, going back and forth to the kitchen eating low-fat breakfast cereal. I ate an 8 oz. bag of pretzels and two pints of low-fat frozen yogurt. I went through the cupboards like a raccoon. Did not exercise today.

After a few nights of late night–snacking, I found myself starting to gain weight again. I was on a limited budget after leaving my husband and only working part-time. Before going to bed one night, I thought to myself, "It's impossible to lose weight when you're on a limited budget." I was eating double portions of those low-fat, portion-controlled foods, and those foods were expensive! Then it struck me, "How did my parents and grandparents get by on a shoestring budget with a house full of children to feed?" I took myself back to my childhood and remembered all the real whole foods that my mother, my Aunt Vernell, and my grandmother used to prepare. Those meals were cooked soulfully and with love, and they satisfied me.

But then I thought about all the time and effort it took to prepare those whole-food meals and I got discouraged again. After working a long hard day, the last thing I felt like doing was cooking a real meal at night. I'm a lazy lima bean when it comes to cooking, and some days it's too much for me even to pop a dinner into the microwave. But I knew in order to change my behavior for a lifetime, I'd have to change my lazy ways too.

And then another lightbulb went off in my head. I thought of a way to have dinner prepared by the time I arrived home from work and have my apartment smelling like someone had made a home-cooked meal especially for me. I ran to the kitchen and dug out my old reliable Crock-Pot. Then I thought about all the meals Mom and Aunt Vernell used to make in my newfound hand-me down treasure and started writing down a list of recipes. I traded in collard greens and hamhocks for "Smoked Turkey Necks and Cabbage," added "Sistah Woman's Naked Stir-Fried Greens" to my repertoire, and turned fried catfish into "oven crispy catfish" with herbs and spices that taste so good it will make your preacher turn his nose up at anything else! And my "Sweet and Savory Sweet Potatoes" will make you want to do more than kiss the cook. (Above recipes found in recipe section.)

I was so excited about the prospect of good, home-cooked food, I couldn't wait till the next morning. I changed out of my night-gown and headed to the nearest twenty-four-hour grocery store at twelve-thirty in the morning. When I got back home I cut up a chicken, some celery, onions, and bell peppers, added a dash of hot pepper and a few herbs for a little kick and let the Crock-Pot do the rest. The next morning I awakened to the smell of heaven. I felt like I was home for Thanksgiving and Mom had been up all night preparing the family feast. The next Saturday I steamed some cabbage, added smoked turkey necks for flavor, and let it just sit cooking until dinnertime. I even made a version of Mom's buttermilk cornbread. My kitchen smelled so good, my dog Heru came in from his usual resting place looking for stray crumbs.

Needless to say, after a full week of eating my glorious whole-food meals, I felt satisfied mentally as well as physically. I did not go back and forth to the kitchen all night looking for something else to eat, my foot was not tapping nervously, and I had wonderful leftovers for lunch. I still popped quick microwave entrées into my food plan a couple of times a week but I did not do this every day like I had in the past. For the first time in my life I did not concentrate on a goal weight or what I would eat as soon as my diet was over. I was more concerned about changing my behavior toward food and exercise. I was loving the process because it gave me peace. I had never experienced the peace, happiness, normal eating, or good mental health that I had now. I was euphoric. I was now in control of what I put in my body. I had stopped dieting! Or so I thought . . .

February 4, 1995

I can't believe I went to the store and brought one of my favorite binge foods home—Haagen-Dazs ice cream! I promised myself I wouldn't bring more than one serving of anything "dangerous" into this apartment. Maybe I shouldn't ever bring home any of my trigger foods (foods that I eat nonstop). But can I live without Haagen-Dazs? Okay, I can. I'm perfectly satisfied with TCBY's low-cal yogurt. In fact, when I ate a few spoonfuls of the Haagen Dazs, it wasn't as good as I remembered. It's too rich and I'm already feeling full. Coming home and putting on my pajamas, surfing the TV channels for Bette Davis or Joan Crawford movies on the classic stations and eating is a sign of relapse for me. I know if I don't find a way to stop, this could be the point of no return. I tried to rationalize how wasteful it was to throw away a pint of expensive gourmet ice cream. Then I heard myself saying out loud, "It's a sin just to throw money away like this," and thought about all the starving people in Africa that Dad used to tell us children about when we didn't finish our dinner. Then I thought about what a sin it was for my hips to look like a tabletop! At 292 pounds, I could have put the TV remote control on my right hip and a cobbler à la mode on the left if my hips had just been a little higher and a little squarer. With that vision in mind I put my wool poncho on over my pajamas and slipped on my boots. I walked to the dumpster and threw in the container of ice cream, all the time visualizing that it was five pounds of fat that I was throwing away.

February 14, 1995

While shopping at Towson Town Center, two saleswomen pissed me off when they told me they did not carry my size in the store. I started craving Popeye's chicken, my old binge hangout. I even drove by the one in Randallstown and parked my car in the parking lot. I sat there for over thirty minutes trying to rationalize why I should have something that would set me up for an all-night binge. I couldn't believe I sat there looking at people eating chicken. The only thing that stopped me from going in was seeing a woman who could barely walk because she was so heavy. It reminded me where I was headed a year ago.

Was throwing that ice cream away worth it? Baby, you'd better believe it! Someone once told me, "If you've started eating something that's loaded with fat and calories and you've already had your share of both today, you have a decision to make. You can either waste it by throwing it away or you can eat it and create waste in you."

I used to try and give extra portions of food away to my neighbors, but then they always complained that I was trying to make them fat. Now I buy trigger foods (cookies, ice cream, potato chips, or chocolate) in the smallest portion possible, but if it's still too much for me to take home, I'll ask the cashier if she/he can take the rest and share it with the other cashiers on their break.

Some of them know my story and will take it without being offended. Others who don't know my story will look at me and say, "I don't believe you'll eat the whole thing. You're not overweight." I just tell them I'm having a bad day and I've been known to eat a whole bag of groceries before arriving home. Most of them laugh along with the customers standing in line and will take me up on my offer of whatever I'm giving away. I'm never too ashamed to be honest about why I will not take more than one portion of a trigger food home. It keeps me on track, allows me to share my story with someone who may be struggling with weight issues, and gives that person an opportunity to try something different. My primary trigger foods are:

> Refined sugar
> White bleached flour
> Any meat full of steroids (think about what consistent high doses of prednisone does to an asthmatic's weight or what high doses of steroids do to athletes)
> Processed white rice
> Processed grain pasta

Wait, wait, don't leave me now. I'm not saying don't eat these foods, I'm just saying I have learned that they can cause problems for me. Some members of my weight-loss workshop have gradually eliminated these foods as part of their new lifestyle, but others have not and are doing well with their weight loss and behavior changes.

What is more important than what I try to eliminate from my food plan is what I have added. Since I have incorporated whole-grain bread, whole-grain pasta, honey, molasses, milled grained or organic natural sugar, fresh fruits and vegetables, brown rice, sea salt, beans/legumes, and fresh fish into my new lifestyle, I eat less but become full much more quickly. Whole foods are high-

quality foods that fill you up quicker than cheap food with no substance. I've also noticed that I have more energy and don't feel as
sluggish or as sleepy after eating a meal. I have severely limited my
dairy and caffeine intake and recently started drinking tap water
with a water filter attached rather than bottled water that has no
flouride to fight against cavities. My acne is clearing up and so are
my blackheads. I no longer suffer from migraine headaches. I got
rid of a benign ovarian cyst without prescription medication or
surgery. My skin and hair have a healthier glow. I feel great, I'm
happy, and I know I'm healthy.

Please don't try to incorporate all of this into your new lifestyle
today. This is a process of *choosing*. I know it can be more expensive to eat this way on a regular basis, but think about the price of
your hypertension, diabetes, migraine, or cardiovascular medications. Think about the price of your smoking or drinking habit.
Think about the price of an emergency-room visit, hospital stay, or
surgery. Think about all the new chain pharmacies popping up in
your neighborhood or favorite grocery or discount store. Now this
is purely a personal opinion, but I think lots of pharmacies in a
small radius represent a sick community. Think about it.

I remember I would cringe at the price of eating healthier whenever my brother Kevin suggested I try a better way of eating. I'd
always cry I was too broke or say that kind of food didn't look or
taste good. I didn't even want to try something healthy or different.
Today I sit back and think about the fat sandwiches that I used to
make. Yep, before eating a piece of beef or pork, I'd trim off the visible fat and layer it on bread covered with mayonnaise and salt.
What could taste worse than that? Don't forget that fat and sugar
are acquired tastes. When people see the way I eat today, they
sometimes call me a health nut. I laugh and think to myself, "It
beats being an unhealthy fool. And what's so nutty about being
healthy? Shouldn't it be the other way around, being an unhealthy
nut?" Remember, this is a process of learning what works and does
not work for you. Be an adventurer! Make a commitment to add or

eliminate something from your diet on a regular basis. Write about how you feel and what, if any, difference it has made.

Close your eyes and imagine being able to walk into a regular-sized clothing store without some obnoxious saleslady saying, "We don't carry your size here." Imagine being able to see your feet without bending over. See yourself not sweating or out of breath when you walk from your car to your front door in seventy-degree weather. Imagine being able to sit down and easily cross your legs at the knee instead of at the ankle. Imagine being able to see and feel your collarbone. Imagine seeing a small space between your upper thighs when you stand with your feet together and look into a full-length mirror. Think of cutting back on, or not having to take, diabetes and hypertension medication. Just imagine actually having the power to add fifteen years to your life! Never in all my wildest dreams did I imagine that I would see any of these things come true for me. But they did, and can come true for you, too.

You're never too old, never too broke, never too pitiful or too obese to change your life. What are you willing to do to become healthy? Think of yourself as a science experiment. Try eliminating those things that come in multiples, like handfuls of crackers or potato chips. If you don't like carrots and celery, don't eat them. If you do go for fried chicken, try getting a two-piece meal instead of the three- (or twelve)-piece deal. Leave something on your plate every time you sit down. Are you really hungry each time you put something in your mouth? Think about what you eat. Use some of my recipes and see if they work for you. Make up some of your own. Exercise. Write in your journal or talk into a tape recorder. Start your own weight loss workshops. Begin to know your body better than any doctor ever could. Build your food plan step by step and brick by brick. There is no penalty for not finishing the construction on time. You are looking for foods that you love to eat, foods that make you feel good, foods that will build a strong, lean foundation to last for a lifetime.

March 6, 1995

Today would have been my brother's thirty-sixth birthday. I'm feeling sad because I miss him so much. It seems like he's only been gone for six months, but it will be two years in June. Kevin would not have wanted me to feel sad today, so I'm going to find a way to remember the good days without getting depressed. Easier said than done. I was on a sales call today sitting in an Ob/Gyn's waiting room for my business appointment until the physician was ready to see me. A lady sitting across from me asked me when my baby was due. When I told her I wasn't pregnant we both wanted to crawl out of the room. I drove around the beltway (1-695) until I talked myself out of going for barbecued spare ribs. Could not come up with three rational reasons why barbecued spare ribs would be good for me physically or mentally. I went home feeling sad and fat. I went to bed early and silently prayed for strength to go on for just one more day.

March 7, 1995

What a difference a day makes. I thank God I didn't drown my sorrows in barbecued spare ribs yesterday. Behavior toward food and exercise was great today! I exercised by walking Heru. I'm joyful and starting to have peace with myself. Today, after listening to CeCe Winans sing "Alone in the Presence," I felt like I could jog to D.C. and back. I have so much energy I took the stairs in most of the office buildings where I had business today. I was hungry at 10 A.M. and stopped to eat my lunch. At first I felt guilty for eating lunch so early. But I'm trying to eat only when I'm hungry. While eating I panicked thinking what would happen if got hungry around 2 P.M. I didn't pack enough food! I thought about all the fast-food restaurants that were lined up on Route 40. I didn't know if I could trust myself going into one of those fast-food chains without ordering greasy foods, and questioned if I was setting myself up for a binge. I thought about foods that still tasted good and then thought of all the places that would sell roasted-turkey sandwiches, baked or grilled chicken-breast sandwiches, or fresh salads. I was afraid of what the smell of onion rings and fries would do to my senses, so I *mentally* choose Subway and *mentally* placed an order that would be satisfying—without all the grease—just in case I needed to stop on the way home. Being prepared is half the battle!

But hey, girlfriend, there's more to this than just food . . .

7

I CAN'T EXERCISE BECAUSE . . .

*T*here's also the second component of weight loss—EXERCISE! I know this is the one thing you were praying I wouldn't mention. Look at it this way, girlfriend. You have your food bricks in place, your emotional windows are open and clean, but you need some electricity in that new body. And that electricity is exercise. You're not there yet, but stick with me and I promise you will consider exercise a gift that you give yourself every day. Let me tell you how powerful a regular exercise regime can be. Days when I don't have the best day in terms of eating *but* I still continue to exercise, my weight stays the same. Days when I *don't* exercise and *don't* have the best day of eating, I gain weight. Days when I eat right and exercise, I tend to lose weight over a period of time. The two components—eating right and exercising on a regular basis—go hand in hand. You must do both if you want to be successful in not only losing weight but, more important, keeping the weight off!

I'll never forget when I first decided finally to start exercising. I went to join a gym. But after overhearing one of the members say to her girlfriend, "If I ever get that big, just shoot me," I left. I felt hurt, angry, and ashamed all at once. I wanted to go back home, eat, and go to bed. But I knew once I got to the bottom of that Haagen-Dazs carton, my problem would still be there. So the next day when I arrived home from work, I bundled up and went for a walk with my dog Heru. My plan was to walk halfway down Kenilworth Drive. But after ten minutes, my lower back began to ache and my knees hurt. Even though it was cold outside, I could feel the sweat running down my back and cleavage. The dog walked too fast and made matters worse. "I can't do it," I thought, "my back and knees hurt too much." I felt like I was going to die from a heart attack because my chest was burning like a furnace out of control. Still, I knew I couldn't give up on exercising like I had done in the past, especially since I wanted to lose over a hundred and fifty pounds. I needed exercises that (number 1) I could do, (number 2) would burn the fat, and (number 3) would tone my skin to minimize sagging. I went to my neighborhood library and read every fitness magazine I could find. I found my answer to getting in shape right there in black and white. I also found a few places that sold sportswear for plus-size women (sports bras, T-shirts, leggings, et cetera). Decent Exposures (1-800 505-4949), Enell Sports Bras (1-800 828-7661), and Danskin Plus (1-800 288-6749). Here is my journal entry for that evening.

March 8, 1995

> While kick-boxing, in-line skating, jogging, and spin-cycling are all fine and dandy for the skinny minis, these are *not* the exercises for me right now. Lord, I know I said I would stop the negative self-talk, but I have a need to get rid of my thunder thighs, fat back, onion butt, Santa stomach, and chicken-wing arms! A lady at the library was kind enough to tell me about exercise videos that I could check out for only fifty

cents. There were videos designed for two-hundred-plus-pound women. I also read about an aqua class available at the local YMCA that was designed especially for guess who— two-hundred-pound women. I can do some toning exercises on the floor right in the comfort of my own apartment. I also learned that I was wearing the wrong shoes for walking and had the wrong attitude. I'm not ready for speed-walking, but I can pace myself by using my Walkman and listening to my favorite slow jams. I can also add ten minutes every week to my walk instead of feeling like I have to walk half a mile. On Friday nights, instead of feeling sorry for myself because I don't have a date, I'm turning my apartment into a discotheque. ("Hey, party over here!").

In my weight-loss workshops I have heard every excuse in the book for not exercising. And all I have to say is that unless you are totally paralyzed, there are NO excuses. I recommend aqua classes for my ladies who have trouble walking because they are either too heavy or have knee or back problems. Water relieves the pressure from the joints while at the same time it provides one of the best cardiovascular workouts around. Okay, I know there are some sisters out there who can't swim or are too embarrassed to wear a bathing suit or don't want to mess up that fancy do. Don't worry, you can stay in the shallow end of the pool and work just as hard. When you are finally ready to venture to the deep end, you can always wear braids or go natural. I had to give up the perm and go natural because I was letting my hair get in the way of my becoming healthier. I had to make a decision: "Do I want to be buried early because I choose to stay at 292 pounds but have a fly hairdo while they lower me into the ground?" Or "Do I want to find an alternative to a fly hairdo that will allow me to become healthy and fabulous?" That's why I choose braids. And about that bathing suit, well, it's up to you how much you want to get to the other side of the bulge.

And if water is really not your thing, then find out what is. Go for a walk, sign up for a yoga class, rent an exercise video—just find some way to move that adds value to your daily routine. Don't expect to become Donna Richardson overnight. You won't, but what you will become is more secure in your ability to do something good for yourself.

Traditionally, Friday was my time to unwind, order takeout from my favorite rib joint, and make a mad dash to Blockbuster's before all the new releases were gone. This would take my mind off my weight and my finances until Monday rolled around. After a few weeks of exercising, though, I was getting used to moving my body, and after one of my home-cooked Crock-Pot meals I would imagine that I had a date to go see Al Jarreau, Take 6, or Maxwell. I would put their music on, or maybe a little Tina Turner or Prince, and dance the night away. If I had a bad day, sometimes I'd light candles, turn off all the lights, and sink into a warm bubble bath. Peabo Bryson, James Ingram, Jeffrey Osborne, Dianne Reeves, Sade, Nina Simone, and the music of Patti LaBelle would help kiss away the pain, but even then the urge to move was stronger than the urge to cry. One night when I thought I was ready to have that good cry, I found myself jumping out of the tub and dancing butt-naked to a Stevie Wonder tune. Something big was happening in my life.

I couldn't rely on my girlfriends to be exercise buddies—they always fizzled out with excuses. I also needed to do lots of different things so I wouldn't get bored. On cold winter mornings, when I would hear the wind racing around my building, I would sink back in bed and pull the covers over my head. Ugh, I knew that spring was a few months away and I couldn't keep hibernating under the covers just because I didn't want to walk by myself anymore. So, on Saturday mornings I started mall-walking with the retired folks. Before I knew it, I had a few sugar daddies wanting to take me to breakfast after walking around the mall. I was flattered, but I hadn't come to the mall to eat. One day while I was walking I passed a store called Successories. This particular store sold motivational and inspirational items—cards, pictures, music, coffee mugs, et cetera. One card in particular, a picture of a lion lying in some tall grass, with a gazelle standing off in the background looking at the lion, caught my eye. The card read:

THE ESSENCE OF SURVIVAL

"Every morning in Africa, a gazelle wakes up. It knows it must run faster than the fastest lion or it will be killed... Every morning a lion wakes up. It knows it must outrun the slowest gazelle or it will starve to death. It doesn't matter whether you are a lion or a gazelle... when the sun comes up, you'd better be running."

I put this card on top of my alarm clock and it's the first thing I see when I want to press the snooze button. This little card rejuvenates me on those mornings when I don't want to exercise (and yes, that still happens). It makes me realize that I want to do more than just survive. I want to feel good and respect myself—now and always.

By July I had lost forty pounds. For me this was a turning point—not just physically but spiritually. For the first time I embraced exercise and nothing got in the way of my daily workout. I was speed-walking now and would put RuPaul's *Supermodel* (a song) on my Walkman and visualize myself as a model swaying my fit body down the runway in Milan, Italy. One very warm Baltimore morning I started out as usual with Heru, and before I knew it I had gone past my usual three miles and had done an extra four miles. I had just experienced my first natural high. As I turned around to head home, I found myself walking faster and faster, not wanting the high to end. I was finally forced to stop when my faithful Heru lay down and refused to take another step. He looked up at me from underneath the shade of a tree as if to say, "Have you lost your damn mind? Do you realize what the heat index is today?" I felt horrible and tried to flag down a cab. They all whizzed by me—the crazy lady with a leash in her hand and a dog looking like it was going into cardiac arrest. We finally got home, but that day Heru taught me an important lesson about myself. I needed to find a balance in order to avoid trading in one addiction for another.

That same evening I was going to see friends and co-workers at a party. They had not seen me since the first of the year. I was looking good and feeling good in what I was wearing. I could look myself in the mirror again because I was loving me. I put on the song that I played each morning, "I'm Gonna Make You Love Me," by Diana Ross and The Temptations. My heart fluttered with excitement as I stared at my reflection, embraced myself, and sang out loud. I carefully applied the makeup I had avoided for so long because I simply did not feel beautiful. As I sang even louder, Heru appeared at my side, frantic with excitement, wagging his tail. I told him I loved him, too, and tried holding back my tears of joy. I didn't want my mascara to run. I had to make my grand entrance and show everyone the fabulous new me.

July 14, 1995

> People who hadn't seen me since last year didn't recognize me. I had to reintroduce myself all evening. Everyone's mouth dropped open as I told them who I was. It felt wonderful! I liked the way people responded to me and I like the way I look and feel. Now I understand why women with good bodies stay on top of their weight—it's not only powerful but they value themselves, and I haven't for so long. I had forgotten how wonderful it feels.

I do a little bit of everything now. I learned to swim so I could move to aqua jogging. I picked up boxing and spin-cycling classes and step aerobics. I even started taking ballet lessons again. Three days a week at 6 A.M. you can find me at (my local gym's) basic training class. This is a military/boot-camp-style workout with former Navy hospital corpsman Cliff Denby and former Air Force M.P. Pat Emery. Rain or shine, these gentlemen lead our class through a workout that guarantees results. Of course, you have to be committed, too. This is by far the most intensive workout I've ever experienced. Just when I think I can't go on anymore, Cliff always says something to motivate me to keep on going, like, "Hey, you're not paying me to walk. JOG! No walking in my class!"

What I love most about this course is the variety. We never do the same routine twice, and each day there is a new challenge. Sometimes we'll jog and stop periodically to do calisthenics. Cliff and Pat always find the biggest hills for us to run up and down. Then, just when I think we're through, they will find an enormous high school stadium full of bleachers to run up and down, then head us back, jogging all the way, to finish our workout in the pool.

Lord knows there are days I want to quit and never return, but I don't. I just keep going. I'm not a long-distance runner by any stretch of the imagination, but just knowing that Cliff and Pat do this rigorous workout with our class in the morning and then again in the evening helps me to push on for another day. When Pat leads the group for a jog, I look at him and can visually see what I have lost. I lost what he weighs, minus three pounds! Some days that's the only thing that keeps me going. I'm not always at the front of the pack with the joggers on our long run, but I'm never at the back of the pack. I always keep in mind the picture that hangs over my bed: *Determination*—"The Race Is Not Always to the Swift . . . But to Those Who Keep on Running."—Corporate Impressions, Successories.

Next summer I may learn to row on a crew team. Maybe I'll train for a race or take up horseback riding or join a softball league. Who knows? It's a big world out there, ladies, and the possibilities are endless. Just think about where I was a few years ago. I never envisioned moving and challenging myself like this. It doesn't matter whether you want to lose five pounds or three hundred pounds. Visualize what you want for yourself and go for it.

Exercise—Medication for the Mind, Body, and Spirit

In years past when I would watch the Olympics, I would marvel at all the hard work and effort it took to become a champion. When the games were over I'd swear I'd start eating right and start exercising again. After two weeks of overdoing exercises that weren't right for me in the first place and jump-starting my broomstick because I was becoming an evil, miserable witch on diet number 219, I'd put a halt to my champion path. When you truly decide to cause a change in your life you can't do things the way you've done them in the past and expect different results. I had to start thinking and behaving like a champion. What about you? Are you ready for a change?

Find an Exercise You Will Enjoy and Adjust Your Attitude

I finally had to put a stop to finding excuses why I couldn't exercise. At 292 pounds, any exercise that I did consistently would help me to lose weight. I knew I had to find time in my day to work toward a full sixty minutes of exercise. They say you're supposed to do at least thirty minutes of aerobic activity at least three days a week to reap the benefits. But I had to do what I could at almost three hundred pounds and build from there. Nobody is at the same fitness level, so everyone has a different starting point. I also had to find an exercise that I would enjoy doing consistently. I had to be prepared at some point to push myself out of my comfort zone and go to a higher-intensity level to continue to lose weight. Just like you would never dream of letting your child stop his learning process at a certain grade level, you shouldn't stop increasing your level of growing stronger and leaner, either. Think hard about what you will do and can do now to put some electricity into your body. Don't let family, work, or being too tired be your excuse for not starting an exercise routine today.

Exercising gives me energy, strength, confidence, and peace. A good workout helps me to sleep soundly at night and allows me to eat what I want within reason. I am no longer limited. I am limitless!

There are three things you should do before starting any exercise program, even walking.

1. Consult with your physician
2. Stretch
3. Drink plenty of water

The first thing you should do is consult with your physician before starting any exercise program. Once you get the go-ahead, take steps to prevent injuries and dehydration. Stretching and drinking water will make an enormous difference on your road to the winner's circle, so pay close attention. I work out a lot but I rarely see anybody stretching or drinking water as they should.

Stretching before and after working out will help reduce injuries. Stretching eases the muscular soreness caused by overdoing any exercise. Stretching allows your body to handle more work and makes your muscles more pliable and supple. S-T-R-E-T-C-H-I-N-G just plain feels good and will give your body a break before you break it!

As an Aquarian, I symbolize the Water Bearer. So as the Water Bearer I want to tell you in very simple terms why drinking water before, after, and during exercise is so important.

Your kidneys can't function properly without enough water, and when they don't work to their full capacity, some of their load is dumped into the liver. One of the primary functions of the liver is to metabolize stored fat into usable energy for the body. But if the liver has to do some of the kidneys' work, it can't operate at its full capacity. As a result, it metabolizes less fat, more fat remains stored in the body and weight loss stops. That information should send you straight to the faucet.

Water suppresses the appetite naturally. Drinking plenty of water is the best treatment for fluid retention because if the body gets too little water, it perceives this as a threat to survival and begins to hold on to every drop. Water is stored in the outside cells and shows up as swollen feet, legs, and hands. Diuretics offer only temporary solutions and force out stored water along with some essential nutrients. Again, the body perceives a threat and will replace lost water at the first opportunity, forcing the condition quickly to return and creating a vicious cycle. The best way to overcome the problem of water retention is to give your body what it needs—plenty of water. Only then will stored water be released.

If you have a constant problem with water retention, excess salt may be the culprit. Your body will tolerate sodium only in certain concentrations. The more salt you eat, the more water your system retains to dilute it. Getting rid of excess salt is easy—just drink more water. As the water is forced through the kidneys, it takes any excess sodium with it.

Water helps maintain proper muscle tone and aids muscles with their natural ability to contract and expand by preventing dehydration. Water helps to reduce the sagging skin that usually follows weight loss (shrinking cells are buoyed by water, which plumps the skin and leaves it clear, healthy, and resilient). Water helps rid the body of waste. During weight loss, the body has a lot more waste to get rid of—all that metabolized fat has to have someplace to go! Water helps relieve constipation. When the body gets too little water, it siphons what it needs from internal sources. The colon is one primary source and the result is constipation. When enough water is put back into the body, normal bowel function usually returns.

Overweight people simply need more water than their thin counterparts. Heavier people have bigger metabolic loads, and water is the key to fat metabolism, kidney, liver, and colon function—hence the overweight person needs more water.

How much water should you drink? On average, a person

should drink eight 8-ounce glasses of water every day. That's just about two quarts. But the overweight person needs one additional glass for every twenty-five pounds of excess weight. For instance, I was 157 pounds overweight. Divide 157 by 25 and you get 6.28, or about six more glasses of water that I needed every day. The amount of water you drink should also increase if you exercise briskly or if the weather is hot and dry. Let's face it, it's really hard to drink too much water!

My doctor told me a story to drive home the point about drinking water. After giving a woman a complete medical examination, the doctor explained his prescription. "Take the green pill with a glass of water when you wake up. Take the blue pill with a glass of water after lunch. Then, just before going to bed, take the red pill with a glass of water." "Exactly what is my problem, Doctor?" the woman asked. "You're not drinking enough water."

Okay, I'm going to give you a chance to stop here if you want to because I'm going to get very specific about the exercises I did, and I'm going to be talking about weights and abductors and stationary bikes and push-ups and the rectus abdominus, and all sorts of other things. You may not be ready to spend time here just yet, but I promise you are going to have to come back here sooner or later.

——————Skip for now.
——————I've got my workout clothes on already.
——————Watch out, Jackie Joyner-Kersee,
   here I come!

I love being outside, so walking was where I started. And even though I do lots of other things, it is still my favorite form of exercise. Walking is highly aerobic and works every part of your body. It's free, uncomplicated, and there is no expensive equipment to buy or to take up room in your house. Just put one foot in front of the other and go! Walking produces few injuries and places minimal stress on the joints. Initially I had problems with shinsplints, but after I learned to stretch before and after my workout and to buy good walking shoes, my shinsplints disappeared. If there's still a problem, stop, contact your doctor, and employ RICE—Rest, Ice, Compression, Elevation. Walking with good posture and breathing correctly was the key to helping me stay injury-free.

As my weight dropped and my fitness level began to improve, so did the intensity of my walks. After a year of walking I was getting bored and my body was getting used to doing the same sixty-minute exercise five days a week, so I started alternating my days of walking with riding my stationary bike and using light weights to build muscle and burn fat. When I walked I chose routes with hills that pushed my commitment and me. Anytime I started getting a little sore in new areas, I knew my weight would drop again. Change your routine if you want to continue to change your body. If you aren't getting the results you want, then you have to challenge yourself to do something different. It's human nature to stick to the same exercise and not move to a different-intensity level. This is also the point where you stop losing weight and get discouraged. Don't give up! Just give up on staying in a rut with the same old exercise routine. Exercise is a gift you can give yourself every day.

Walking does more than just exercise my body. Walking, particularly in a beautiful place, helps me to clear my mind and reflect and make decisions that give me peace of mind. Walking calms me down when I'm angry, energizes me when I'm bored, and renews me when I'm exhausted after a day's work. I lost seventy-five percent of my weight by walking and light weight lifting. I started off walking twice a week for only ten minutes because that's all I could do. Then I slowly added ten minutes each week and began walking faster. My favorite music in my Walkman motivated me to walk at a certain pace and keep walking for my allotted time. Go at your own pace when you begin, but remember that a champion in training always has a vision and will push to the next level. If walking really is too tough on your joints right now, see if you can find a pool and walk back and forth in the shallow end. At the very least start stretching.*

On to the exercises I did in my apartment with just the TV and the dog for company. Let's talk a minute about the muscles you will be working. Did you know that your buttock is the largest muscle in your body? No big surprise, huh? Your buttocks help you jump and climb hills and stairs. Along with the buttocks there is the thigh with its four components—outer thigh, inner thigh, quadriceps, and hamstring. I have a tendency to carry a lot of weight in my hips and thighs, and this was the most challenging part, and the last part, of my body to change.

Your outer thigh, the abductor, is the fattest part of the hip. It helps you move sideways, rotate your hip outward. The inner thigh, the adductor, runs from inside the hip. If strong enough, the inner thigh muscles can crush a cantaloupe or small watermelon. Try in-line skating, or horseback riding, or riding a motorcycle if you have any doubts about how much you need to work this muscle.

The quadriceps are the four muscles at the front of the thigh and they work together to operate the knee as you walk. If your knees hurt, these are the muscles to work on. Remember always to consult with your physician any time you experience a persistent pain.

Your hamstrings are the three muscles at the back of your thigh and they work opposite the quadriceps. This is a muscle you hear a lot about, particularly among professional athletes. Hamstrings are prone to pulls and soreness, and you can never stretch them

---

* If you have more than a hundred pounds to lose like I did, you may not be able to do some of these exercises. DO NOT GIVE UP! I couldn't even do two pushups when I started. If you can't do the pushups, then stick with the biceps curls. If you can't do the abdominal crunches, then work on your back muscles. Find what you can do and start there.

too much when warming up or cooling down. They also help support your buttock muscle.

And just to round things out, you need to think about the large diamond-shaped muscles at the back of your lower leg—your calf muscles. If you ever pulled one of these, you know you won't be going anywhere for a while. Let's try an exercise that will improve strength and endurance in your lower body before discussing walking more.

Buttocks, Hamstrings, and Quadriceps
While performing this exercise, maintain a stable position of the lower spine throughout, with the heels of your feet in contact with the floor at all times. This exercise can be performed with or without a flex ball.

WITH FLEX BALL: Stand with your back to a wall, 12–14 inches away, feet hip-width apart. Place a flex ball between your lower back and the wall. Move your feet forward, keeping your abs contracted and rib cage lifted, with pelvis in a neutral position. Bend your knees to squat, letting the ball roll up the wall (and your back) until your thighs are parallel to the floor. Don't let your knees move forward beyond your toes. Hold as long as you can. Return to the starting position and repeat.

WITHOUT FLEX BALL: Stand with your back against the wall. Bend your knees, squatting down until your hips are parallel with your knees, and hold as long as possible. Don't let your knees move forward beyond your toes. Return to the starting position and repeat. Try working up to one-to-two minutes while in squatting position.

Now back to walking. I know some days the heat and humidity or the bitter cold is just unbearable. That is when I pull out my stationary bike and turn on the trashiest TV show I can find or read the latest issue of my fitness magazine and indulge in a bit of daydreaming. I have had my bike since 1992, but it didn't get any real use until 1995. In fact, over half the women in my workshops confessed to having treadmills, bikes, and Nordic Tracks that were either gathering dust or clothes. If you are in the market for one, I promise you, this is a piece of equipment that you will find at almost any yard sale. No need to spend a lot of money here, but it sure does come in handy. Stationary cycling is easy and just about injury-free. My hips, thighs, and calves started changing as I increased the tension and the length of time I rode. I increased my riding time exactly the way I did my walking, by adding ten minutes each week until I was up to sixty minutes. My calves got longer and leaner and my hips and thighs got toned. What more can you ask for? On the weekends, when I had time, I added light weights for my upper body, especially those arms and obliques.

Ladies, I never dreamed of seeing my feet again when I reached 292 pounds. But I thank God that today I can! I really had to work on having a positive attitude when it came to my abdominal workout because I had heard all these myths about doing five-hundred-to-a-thousand crunches a day to keep toned and strong.

Waistline

Your waistline is the indentation in the middle of your torso, and genetics help determine its dimensions. Some women have only a little indentation at the waist, while others have classic hourglass figures. You can only narrow your waist by developing strong rectus abdominus and oblique muscles (they wrap diagonally from the spine to the front of your abdomen), and even then your body type will be the final determinant.

The rectus abdominus is one long muscle that runs from the rib cage to the pubic bone. There are no upper and lower abs. When you contract your abs, you involve the entire muscle. Different kinds of exercises stimulate different parts of the muscle, and that is why you hear about upper and lower abs. Don't expect the same muscle definition below your navel as you might higher up because the lower abdominal muscles are longer and would require stimulation involving a movement where the hips would move toward the ribs (that is, a reverse crunch). If you don't do these exercises correctly, you don't eliminate excess body fat, and if you're not genetically predisposed to have a superflat belly, you won't have a washboard stomach. Sorry, that's just one of the facts of life. Fundamentally, women's bodies were designed so their abdomens could expand to carry babies, and not much has changed in that regard since Eve played around in the Garden of Eden. The key to a strong, firm abdominal wall is correct technique, consistency, and, of course, eating right. I thought I knew how to do ab work, but by the time I finished one set I was dripping with sweat and felt like I hadn't done a thing. Learning to feel what position gave me the greatest benefit made a big difference in my workout. It's just like everything else we have talked about—you have to find what works for you.

Try to work up to doing a set of these next exercises two-to-three days a week. Do two sets of one-to-fifteen repetitions, resting thirty seconds between sets. When you can do both sets easily and with good form, progress by adding another set.

Abdominal Crunch

Practice lying on your back in a neutral position with your knees bent and with your feet flat on the floor, hip-width apart. Take a deep breath and as you exhale suddenly stop your air from going out. At this state, your abs should be tight. Continue breathing.

Now place a pad or mat on the floor and lie face-up on the mat, with your feet flat on the floor, hip-width apart, and the top of your head at the mat's edge. Hold the corners of the mat in each hand, with elbows slightly flared, relaxing your head against it. Your mat is your support for your head and neck. You don't have to invest in the latest ab machine because you've just created your own using the mat. Contract your abdominal, inhale, and move your ribs forward, your hips, neck, and shoulders off the floor as you bring your ribs toward your hips, using the mat for support. Begin to exhale just as your shoulders lift off the floor. Take two slow counts to lower yourself to starting position and repeat.

Obliques

When working the obliques, remember you also work them while performing a crunch. Please note that technique is very critical when performing this abdominal exercise. We want to eliminate any risk of placing undue stress on the spine.

On the same mat, lie flat on your back with knees bent. Place your hands behind your head, unclasped, and keep elbows open to the ceiling. In this position lean both legs to one side, while lying slightly on your hip, but note your knees are not to touch the ground. Don't worry if you can't get all of you "over"—just do the best you can. Your shoulder blades should remain flat on the floor. Now tighten your abs and lift your ribs toward your hip in a twisting movement going toward your knees. Return to your starting position, repeat ten-to-fifteen times, rest for thirty seconds, repeat another ten-to-fifteen times, and then turn your torso to the other side and start again. Do what you can. If you can only do five, then fine. Do five for several weeks and then add one or two more lifts. The more you do, the more you can do.

Even though our skin becomes less toned as we age, you can still have firm abs by keeping a check on your body fat and including abdominal strength training in your regular workout routine.

Strength Training for Toning and Losing Weight

Aerobic exercise helps burn calories and revs up your metabolism. But when you add a few strength-training workouts each week, alternating with the days of aerobic activity, you are putting the pedal to the metal. You gain lean body tissue and can actually speed up your metabolism. Remember, the more muscle you have, the more calories you will burn. Don't freak out if the scale shows a weight gain. Instead look at how your clothes are starting to fit you. When I started weight training, I started fitting into smaller sizes even though I had not lost a lot of weight. That's because muscle takes up less room than fat. It never fails—when I am invited to speak at various workshops across the country, someone always asks, "How much do you weigh and what size do you wear?" Although I don't like measuring my weight by a scale, I always do it before I go to speak in front of a group. I just have to have that number ready for them, and I can always use it to make a point. One morning I weighed in at 137 pounds and was sliding into a size 6. When I was asked the inevitable question and I gave my honest, up-to-date answer, I had women screaming! Of course they all wanted to know how, if they weighed less than I did, they were still wearing a size 10 or 12 or maybe even size 14. It's all about body fat! Lean muscle tissue is sleek and mean and makes you look smaller. Heavy, bulky fat is just that—heavy, bulky, and fat.

Now are you ready to lift some light weights? You are not going to be muscle-bound. You are not going to look "unfeminine." You are not going to look like a man. Let's get the facts straight about what strength training can do for you. Lifting weight makes you and your bones stronger and goes a long way toward avoiding osteoporosis later in life.

Lifting weights is an excellent way to prevent injuries because when your muscles are strong, they are simply less prone to injury and stress. Strength training is one of the keys to long-term permanent weight management. Although you can't spot-reduce, you can spot-shape and redesign your proportions. I wanted firmer and shapelier hips, so I started building up my back and shoulders to give my hips a smaller appearance. It turned my heavy, fleshy, soft-pear look into a streamlined, fine, firm, and tight look. Strength training can help improve your muscle-to-fat ratio and increase your metabolism.

You will not begin to see definition, or the outline, of your muscles until you get rid of the thick layer of fat that covers them. You will begin to see some definition when your body fat dips into the

22-to-20 percent range, or after about six weeks of alternate-day strength training. Results will vary, depending on the amount of time and effort you put into your workout, your starting point, and your body type. The more you have to lose, the longer it will take for you to see definition. I never dreamed I would see definition anywhere on my body, but when I did it was a wonderful feeling of accomplishment, so don't give up. And if you still have any doubts about looking muscle-bound, just look at my pictures—I have been strength training for four years now.

Where do you get these weights? Any sporting-goods store will have a variety (shape, color, and size) of weights, or, if you aren't ready to buy anything, roll up a couple of issues of "W" magazine and put a rubber band around them. Find two books. Use two bricks. It doesn't matter, just do it.

Triceps
You'll find your triceps at the back of your upper arm. Strong triceps will help lessen the elbow pain you get from carrying a heavy box or child or a briefcase, or from playing too much tennis. Toning the triceps will help tighten back-of-the-arm flab and increase your upper-body strength.

It's time to get armed and dangerous. If you're like me, you don't want fat chicken wings hanging out of all your sleeveless summer dresses. Give this a good six weeks and you'll see a difference.

Let's start with the triceps, since this seems to be the most neglected and weakest portion on our arm. To prevent the common mistakes of arching your back or leaning your torso, which may happen when doing sitting or triceps extensions, I like to lie in a safe, almost injury-free position that allows me to maintain spinal alignment.

Grab a pair of one-to-two pound dumbbells or a weight that feels comfortable to you and that you can *control*. Lie on your back on a bench or an ottoman or build your own bench with a high-leveled stepper. While lying on your back with knees bent, make sure your feet are flat on the floor and extend your hands, raising dumbbells toward the ceiling with palms facing each other. Now bend your arms at the elbow, lowering the weights toward the side of your head. Note: Where your elbow starts is where it stays. Slowly extend the arms until elbows are straight but not locked and be careful not to overextend the elbow joint. Pause briefly at the top of the movement, then slowly bend the elbows and return to the starting position. Throughout the exercise, remember to keep your abs contracted and your head in line with your spine. Do one-to-two sets of ten reps, working up to fifteen rep sets. When fifteen can be performed with good form, gradually increase the resistance in one-pound increments, to as much as eight pounds per hand. Each time you increase the weight, remember to start with ten reps and work back up to fifteen reps before you increase the weight again. If you experience any pain or discomfort, try using lighter weights or no weight at all until you become stronger.

Biceps
Your biceps are the two muscles in front of your upper arm. Strong biceps make lifting anything easier. Strong biceps are sexy and will look great in that slinky off-the-shoulder summer dress.

Stand with your legs shoulder-width apart, knees slightly bent and arms at your side with your palms facing down. Start off with a two-pound weight in each hand. Keeping your upper arms still and bending at the elbow (remember to keep wrists straight), begin to move the weights by imagining that you are bringing your hands toward your face. Once you reach the top of your movement, *s-q-u-e-e-z-e* your biceps (don't squeeze your hands) Picture yourself as having a walnut in the pit of your arm and you're trying to crack it open. Just as with the triceps, where the elbows start is where they must stay. Do three sets of ten repetitions. Start off with two-pounds weights. When two pounds becomes easy, increase their weight.

Chest (Pectorals and Shoulders (Deltoids)

There are two chest muscles: the pectoral major and the pectoral minor. Both help you push the grocery cart and the lawn mower, or to wrap your arms around that big wonderful brother. Women's pectorals are located right underneath the breasts. Breasts will sag with age, but strong pecs help give a more youthful appearance.

SHOULDERS (DELTOIDS): This muscle sits at the top of your arm and attaches to the upper part of your chest and to your shoulder blade. Strong shoulders help avoid dislocations and assist the chest and back muscles. Want to throw out those shoulder pads? Want to turn a few heads with a strapless evening gown or tube top? Then this is the muscle to work. For those of you with large breasts, working these muscles will take some of the strain off your back and make it easier to move. And for those less well-endowed sisters, definition of these muscles goes a long way toward enhancing Mother Nature.

Modified push-ups are like hitting a home run—they work the triceps, chest, and shoulders. Place your exercise mat on the floor and get into standard push-up position but bend your knees so that they touch the ground and your weight is supported by the upper legs. Keep head and chest lifted and contract the abdominal muscles as you lower your torso toward the floor and exhale. Inhale as you straighten arms and return the chest to starting position. Begin with three sets of five repetitions each. If that is too much for you, start lower and build from your starting point. Work up to twelve-to-fifteen repetitions per set. Allow yourself at least five seconds of rest between sets. Don't get discouraged. When I started out I couldn't complete two sets of five repetitions. It doesn't matter how many you start with, what matters is that you do it and with proper form, keep doing it, and then find yourself doing more.

If you find this exercise too difficult to begin with, the alternative is to use a wall. Stand facing a wall an arm's length away. Place hands flat against the wall, take one step back, move hands down around chest level and a little wider than shoulder width. Keeping abdominals tight, lean your chest toward the wall. Make sure you don't bend at the waist, but move the body as a whole. Return to starting position.

THE PEC FLY (CHEST AND SHOULDER SHAPER): Position yourself on your bench on your back, with your knees bent and feet flat on the floor—feet should be 12–18 inches apart. Using a two- or five-pound dumbbell in each hand, pretend you are wrapping your arms around a barrel as you raise your arms inward and directly above your chest, palms facing forward and about one inch apart. Keep your arms, wrists, and elbows slightly rounded. Slowly lower your arms in an arclike pattern until you feel a gentle stretch across the front of your shoulders—until your elbows are even with shoulder height. Do not let arms drop all the way back toward the floor. Pause and then slowly start the movement again. Make sure to maintain smooth control throughout the arclike movement and be careful not to rely on speed or momentum to raise or lower your arms. Concentrate on using the abdominals to keep your pelvis and torso stable and avoid letting the lower back arch when your arms are in the lowered position. Concentrate on isolating the movement to the shoulder and chest area.

Try one-to three sets of eight reps, working up to sets of twelve reps each. Do this exercise two-to-three times per week. When twelve repetitions can be performed with good form, gradually increase the resistance in one-to-two-pound increments, to as much as fifteen pounds per hand. Each time you increase the weight, begin with eight reps per set, working back up to twelve reps per set before the next weight increase.

Lower and Upper Back (Latissimus Dorsi)

The lower-back muscles run the entire length of your spine to strengthen and straighten it. These muscles are the foundation for much of our bending, lifting, and turning. Many people suffer from back pain. In fact, eighty percent of adults will have back pain at some point in their lives, but much of this suffering is preventable if we maintain a good balance of abdominal and lower-back strength. Strong lower backs are also vital for maintaining good posture.

UPPER BACK (LATISSIMUS DORSI): The largest muscle in the upper body is called the "lat" and runs the entire length of your back from your shoulders to the top of your hips. These muscles do all of the upper-body pulling movements. Strong lats make your hips and waist appear smaller by adding contour and width to your upper body. Golf, rowing, tennis, racquetball, and basketball all make heavy use of lats. Runners and walkers should focus on their lats to help counteract any tendency toward rounded shoulders. Everybody looks good when they stand up straight. Strong lats are another real help for those who carry a lot on the front of their chests!

REVERSE FLY (UPPER BACK): Lie face-down on your bench with legs bent at about ninety degrees. Hold a three-to-eight-pound dumbbell in each hand with elbows bent at about fifteen degrees and arms to each side so the hands are just off the floor with palms facing downward. Contract abdominals to bring spine to a neutral position—your chest will lift slightly off the bench. Lift elbows up and out to your sides as far as they can go without dropping your shoulders. Slowly return your arms to the original position and repeat. Try to do between ten and fifteen repetitions on the first set, then ten-to-fifteen on the second set. Rest sixty seconds between sets. The speed of each movement is three seconds up, hold for a count, then down for five. With concentrated effort and good form, you'll feel all the upper back muscles working. Keep wrists and forearms in line as they work as a single unit. Keep your arms relaxed so you can isolate your shoulder muscles.

PELVIC LIFTS (LOWER BACK STRETCHES): This exercise not only stretches and strengthens your lower back but also works your buttocks, abs, and hamstrings.

Lie on a mat on your back with your knees bent and feet flat on the floor and hip-width apart. Place hands underneath your head. Anchor your back to the floor by pulling your abdominals in toward your spine. Squeeze your buttocks together and lift your hipbones up until your buttocks are about two inches off the floor. Hold a moment and slowly lower and start again. Make sure you do not arch your back off the floor.

Swimming

Thank God for swimming! It was tough losing my last fifteen pounds. In fact, it took me a year to lose the last ten. I thought I was in pretty good shape after jogging, biking, aerobics classes, et cetera. But swimming was a struggle. I could barely do one lap! Swimming is one of the best forms of exercise around because it works so many things at the same time. Swimming uses both your upper and lower body, burns tons of calories, and is easy on your joints. I'm still not the best swimmer in the world, so sometimes I'll just work out in the shallow end of the pool with water dumbbells. By doing my strength training submerged in water, I have built more muscle because the simple motion of the water forces my trunk, abdominal, and lower-back muscles to work harder at stabilizing my body and keeping me upright. According to Mary Sanders, M.S., Education Director for Speedo International and adjunct faculty member at the University of Nevada, Reno, "Since strength-training machines do most of the stabilizing for you, the stabilizing muscles may not work as hard or as long on land as they do in the water." And if you don't believe your gym workout can compare to a cardio pool workout, check this. Research suggests that you can burn as many or more calories in the water as on solid ground. Compare the following:

Activity	Kilocalories burned per minute*
Water—aquatic strength training	5.7–6.5
Land—Circuit weight training	5.1–6.1
Water—Deep-water walking	8.8
Land—Walking (normal pace)	4.7
Water—Deep-water running	11.5
Land—Running (11-minute mile)	8.0

*Source: Courtesy of Len Kravitz, Ph.D., University of Mississippi in Oxford.

So for anyone trying to get rid of those last fifteen-to-twenty pounds, try a pool.

Unfortunately, research also suggests that one of the drawbacks for people who carry excess body fat is that swimming may not be very effective. It seems the more fat you have on your body, the more you float and the less you work. I say take this with a grain of salt. If you like being in the water and it will get you moving, then go for it. You're not going to be carrying all that excess weight forever!

All the exercises I have talked about are the same ones I did on a regular basis to lose over one hundred and fifty pounds. I didn't have a personal trainer, I didn't go to a gym, and I didn't have a lot of expensive equipment at home. I've become a certified personal trainer, and have started training clients in my weight-loss workshop. I may be one of the only personal trainers with fat stretch marks. Pretty good advertisement for a lifestyle change, I'd say! I'm so grateful for all the opportunities that have come my way and now I'm giving something back.

—

I love changing my exercise routine and am always looking for something different and challenging. Please remember I didn't just start off doing these exercises—I had to work slowly on each one of them. It doesn't matter what you weigh or how old your are; you can do some form of exercise. Exercising is simply part of my life and something I do automatically, just like I automatically brush my teeth in the morning, I automatically think about what exercise routine I'll do that day. Exercise is my lifeline for continued success.

8

GETTING HONEST TO BE FREE

*T*his is confession time. As an obese woman I was the biggest liar in the world. Taking my sins to the altar on Sunday was a joke. Who did I think I was fooling by promising to start fresh on Monday with diet number 200. And who was I making that promise to? I knew deep within that just laying my troubles on God's doorstep was not enough. I needed more than just talking the talk. I needed to walk the walk. I needed to be honest with myself in every way, every day.

Keeping a daily journal is an important outlet for a very emotional subject—fat. I did not weigh 292 pounds just because my stomach was growling. I weighed 292 pounds because I had no place to take my pain, frustration, sadness, or fear. Just as I had to learn what foods worked and didn't work for me, I had to open the windows of my soul so my emotions could fly free instead of sticking to my thighs and stomach. I had to eat in the now, not in the hurt of yesterday or the possibilities of tomorrow. My journal was and is my greatest source of comfort. It records my life, it helps me to remember, it keeps me honest about *why* I eat.

Just like most of you, I've been on and off various weight-loss programs. Almost all of these programs recommend some form of journal writing. I absolutely fought tooth and nail against writing down my feelings. Instead, I would write down what I was eating on bits and pieces of paper—nothing permanent, nothing I could *use.* I would usually start my diets on Monday, so that morning I could write down what I had eaten. By noon I only wrote down half of what I had really eaten, and by evening I had stopped writing altogether because I wanted to forget my binge. I never wrote down my feelings because I was in denial—about everything. Asking me, at 292 pounds, to write down everything I put into my mouth and why I ate it was a joke. After a while I simply refused to acknowledge that I was in pain. I always pretended that everything was okay, when the whole world could just look at my swollen body and see that I wasn't.

The last diet program I was involved in—before I stopped dieting for good—was a liquid fasting program run by a physician and a nutritionist. This time I did write down everything I ate. I thought maybe if I mustered up the courage to write about my binges, then somehow whoever read it could help me and the weight would start to melt away. It was horrible and hard, but I did it anyway. I had just had one of my worst binges, and this is what my food diary looked like:

Breakfast	Calories	Fat grams
4 slices of bread	280	4
1 lb. of cured bacon	763	66
2 fried eggs (large)	182	14

Lunch	Calories	Fat grams
.99-cent bag of		
Utz potato chips	525	31

Dinner	Calories	Fat grams
2 very large porterhouse steaks	1554	112.8
Haagen-Dazs 1 pint (vanilla)	1240	84
1 Marie Calendar peach cobbler	1440	72

Total Calories—5,984

Total Fat Grams 383.8

Note—it takes 3,500 calories to gain 1 pound

The group leader looked over all of our journals and commented briefly on everyone's week without revealing whose journal she was reading. When she got to mine she stated emphatically, "This person clearly did not eat this much and has calculated the calories and fat grams wrong." I couldn't believe my ears. Here I was sitting in a roomful of obese people, some weighing over four hundred pounds, and she couldn't believe someone ate this way! I knew the calories and fat grams were accurate because I read the nutritional labels on the back and used my trusty calculator and all of my calorie and carbohydrate counter books. Who needed this!

For once I was brave enough and honest enough to write down something I was ashamed of and this was the response I got? After class I went to the instructor and told her that my calculations were correct and that I did eat everything I had written down. She was shocked and recommended that I make an appointment to see her to talk about what I was eating. I didn't make an appointment because I had already spent so much on the program and didn't have the additional money to pay for an hour session with her—especially now that I knew she was clueless. I did try journal writing many other times, but I was never honest enough with myself about what was really bothering me. I knew if I *honestly* wrote about my feelings, then I would have to have some sort of reaction to the horror on the paper. Then I would have to do something about it, which meant change, and that scared me even more.

But in 1994, on New Year's Eve, as I prayed in the safety of my pew, with my size-22 skirt cutting my waist, I knew I *had* to make a change. I was in crisis. I was tired of living but more afraid of taking my own life. How and where would I begin to share my feelings of fear, hurt, shame, self-pity, and anger? What would move me from wallowing in the self-pity and denial that had me tipping the scales at 292 pounds and busting out of a size-22 skirt?

It was really very simple. The vehicle that would motivate me, support me, and allow me to lose weight was an 8½-by-10 notebook. It would move me to a place of acceptance, respect, and acknowledgment. My journal would become my safe haven, my therapist's couch, my best friend, my sanctuary, my communion with God. I started writing. I was terrified. Why would it be any different this time? *Maybe because I was doing this for me and no one else.*

I wrote in my journal almost daily. I wrote about my day and how I interacted with people. I wrote down my feelings of pain, the source of the pain, and how I dealt with the pain *and* the source. I also wrote down my feelings of happiness. I started tracking my eating patterns and triggers and made up action plans on how to avoid a bad eating situation the next day. I wrote down when I exercised and for how long, what I ate, when I ate, how much I ate, and where I ate it. My journal did not judge me, it did not make me right or wrong, it did not say I was bad or good. It was simply *my* journal.

Writing helped me to become honest again. Writing allowed me to cry, scream, and feel the pain I had suppressed for so long. Writing helped me to grieve and, finally, to heal.

As a binger I had learned to lie about so many things. For years I lied about being okay, when I really felt depressed and didn't care if I lived or died. I lied about my marriage when I knew it was doomed from the start. I lied about my brother's health. I hid the amount of food I ate. I lied about the amount of money I spent on my food addiction. I lied about almost everything.

But with my journal I was free to be honest. I was able to write, freely and openly, about what was on my mind. I wasn't judged, criticized, or shunned. Some days I wrote pages, sometimes just a sentence or two, and sometimes, very rarely, nothing at all.

As I started to write seriously, I felt a sense of relief and realized I was finally letting go of the heavy burdens I had kept inside me for thirty-three years. Now I know why I rebelled against this process for so many years. Journal writing is painful if you write honestly. There were days when I could not remember certain events, but then, usually that night, my dreams would bring the dark memories to the surface. The next day I would be left to face the pain and work through it. But once I started, once I knew that the other side was *always* better, there was no NOT facing the pain.

I learned volumes about myself. I learned that instead of speaking my mind I silenced myself with food just like I had silenced my first scream when my grandfather walked in on me in the bathroom. Food was punishment and reward. It was anger and fear and despair. It was everything except what it is supposed to be— nutrition. It's hard for me to believe sometimes that such a simple act as writing has had such a profound effect on my life. Years of dieting made me fatter, and years of journal writing, just telling the truth, did the opposite. It's amazing that when you finally start working on the inside, the outside responds so readily. The weight of the world seemed lifted from my mind. My spirit was freed to soar and grow.

Journal writing helped me realize that food was not my problem—it was only a symptom of many problems. After weeks of being on starvation diets, being thin never miraculously made me happy. For years I had placed so many limitations on myself because of my weight. It was like living in a prison without locks. Releasing my thoughts on a piece of paper forced me to stand outside myself and look objectively at who I was and what I had created in my life. After a few months of progressive journal writing, I went back and reread some of my early entries. It was then that I decided to redirect and change the course of my life. It was like reading a book with no ending—having the power to create the ending that I wanted.

Journal writing has given me faith, vision, passion, and a tremendous sense of purpose. Whenever I feel out of balance, the one thing I can count on to bring me serenity and peace is writing in my journal. God is present on every page and I know he will not fail me.

When I started my journal, it was difficult to reread the sometimes dark, ugly moments in my life. But that simple act has led me to a greater personal and spiritual development. Reviewing my journals, especially as I started on this book, was like looking at my life on a large movie screen. The bingeing scenes were especially painful—it was like watching myself voluntarily commit a slow suicide. At the same time, it was a challenge. A challenge to reclaim my life and dare to dream what had never seemed possible.

Did I truly have the power to change my life-denying habits after bingeing for twenty-seven years? For so many years I'd felt purposeless, weak, and inadequate. How would I lift the clouds of depression that had followed me for years? The only way I knew to escape from my old life was to write. Some days it seemed so painful, but I knew that if I avoided writing out the pain I would find another way to release it—and that release almost always led to bingeing. I would write and cry until my eyes were swollen shut; I refused to let food temporarily and falsely comfort me. Those were days when I could look at myself in the mirror the next morning, knowing I had made it through another day without using food as anything but nutrition. Writing helped me to commit to a new way of living. Whatever I wrote down on paper I claimed as my challenge for the day. If anyone hurt me or made me angry, I wrote about it, slept on it, and vowed to do something about it. I no longer allowed people to take advantage of me or run over me. For too many years I had allowed people to treat me badly and then used food to make myself feel better. When I initially decided to stand up for myself, I was so full of aggression that I went to the opposite spectrum and returned the bad treatment. Now I try not to react. I think, I write, I pray, and I act accordingly.

The days I didn't write were the days I had trouble with my food. But as I began to put the missing pieces of my life together, I found the voice I had lost as an eight-year-old child. I was able to grow and love myself again.

Journal writing allows me to work on my excess baggage while taking time to reflect and contemplate ways to avoid repeating the past. I never knew how to nurture or care for myself and never allowed anyone to give me the love that I longed for. As a result I've attracted men in my life who were never able to commit to me or give me the unconditional love I so wanted and deserved.

Journal writing helped me examine the friends I attracted to my life. I decided to write about each one of my friends and whether or not they were to remain in my life. For many years I allowed anyone to be my friend, but now I know that I get to choose. I need support, love, generosity, and compassion. Some of those who I called friends are no longer. It's amazing how once you start taking care of yourself, how once you become mentally and physically fit, then those unhealthy friends of yesteryear start to disappear. The friends I choose now, men and women, enrich my life and allow me to enrich theirs.

I realize that journal writing does not work the same way for everyone. Just the words "journal" and "write" are scary for some people. Some women in my workshops find talking into a tape recorder helps them to deal with the pain and hurt. Others have found the need for professional counseling. Many have used a combination of self-examination and professional help. Use what works for you, but use something. Start slowly. You didn't become fat, afraid, or dishonest overnight, and you won't be thin tomorrow. Take your time. Congratulate yourself. You've started your building program with foods that work for you and now it is time to put in some clean, sparkling windows. Take in the view to a rich new life—it looks pretty good!

September 15, 1995

> I can finally see for the first time that I am actually smaller. I don't feel huge anymore. But I'm afraid to lose more weight even though I want and need to lose more. The men are starting to take notice and give me more attention and this scares me and makes me nervous. The women are getting cattier because they are feeling threatened by me. If they only knew how I hated the attention from men. My naturally bubbly personality is starting to surface again and I realize for the first time that most people are unhappy and get mad at you for being happy. I'm being accused of being phony and hear things like "What are you so happy about?" I don't want to crumble and conform like I used to before because I'm sick of being a coward. I don't want to go back to thoughts of being buried in a piano case and being in a state of constant dark depression. I'm tired of living my life to please others. I don't want to play the "Aunt Jemima" role anymore! I'm not this strong African-American woman who is the caretaker, nurturer, and healer to other people. I'm a delicate flower that sometimes breaks in the wind, too. I will

deal with men giving me attention again and the unhappy people in a different way: Feel the fear but do anything but eat over it. Get over it, and to hell with any sister who hates me for getting fit, fine, and fabulous! Never again will I allow anyone, ever, to still my joy!

9

BEEN THERE, DONE THAT

*M*y path from 292 pounds to 133 pounds was full of left turns, right turns, and an occasional U-turn. There are no straight lines on the road map to good health. You will have lapses and relapses. Forgive yourself and move quickly to get back on track. Determine what caused your derailment and implement a plan of action to overcome the next potential obstacle. Look in the mirror and say, "I LOVE YOU." Write in your journal about what happened.

We've all been on all the fad diets and weight-loss programs. Most of them worked, but only in the short term. I finally understood that the only way for me to lose weight and keep it off was first to start working on what was eating me, to stop dieting and start exercising. It took me thirty-four years and at least ten different diets to realize finally that I was not getting any thinner.

Diets I lost and gained weight on over the years

Liquid fast • Cabbage-soup diet • No-fat diet
Pills • Grapefruit diet • Tea diet

Hypnosis   •   Protein Diet   •   Eat all you want until 12 noon
Weight-loss programs   •   Low-/No-carbohydrate diet

We have all "been there, done that" and just grown fatter. Now is the time to continue the lifestyle change that you have started to put in place. I'd like to introduce you to Marilyn McCraven, who was one of the very first members of my weight-loss workshops. As I told you in Chapter 4, I started my own weight-loss workshops after everyone started coming to me asking for advice on how I managed to lose 157 pounds. Initially, I started out with just a few people in my apartment, cooking my favorite recipes and sharing with them how I stopped dieting and finally started to make a lifestyle change. But as my story began to appear in major magazines, the size of my group became too large for my small apartment. I moved my workshop to a gym where I now currently hold workshops and train clients as a personal trainer.

Marilyn McCraven

Age: 44—Married
Mother of two sons, 9 years and 12 years
Starting weight: 278 pounds.
Height: 5'3"
Weight lost to date: 70 lbs.
Inches lost: 54

Marilyn has been married for fifteen years, and losing weight has been a constant struggle. I met Marilyn when she used to be a reporter for a major newspaper. I wanted to spread the word about my workshop so I called the newspaper and spoke with Marilyn about my story. She had read about me earlier in *Essence* magazine and was interested in not only doing the story but also wanted to join my weight-loss workshop.

Marilyn's job was both sedentary and stressful. She would sit for hours at the computer writing stories and conducting telephone interviews. Breakfast was sporadic, maybe yogurt or cold cereal with fruit. She often worked through lunch and would then find herself picking up a quick bite to eat at fast-food drive-throughs while taking her sons to soccer practice. After finally getting home for the evening, she would eat her largest meal around 8 P.M. While her sons bathed and got ready for bed, she would often go back to the kitchen and binge. Like me, Marilyn loves sweets and felt this was her real downfall. After bingeing she would be out of control and depressed. The only time she exercised was when she dieted. As soon as the diets ended, so did the exercising.

A few months later Marilyn joined my weight-loss workshop (August 1997). I gave everyone a blueprint for success and Marilyn ran with it. Marilyn is athletic and used to play intramural basketball and volleyball in high school, so she was no stranger to exercise. The day after her first class she started working out with a personal trainer despite an aching back and knees. Marilyn soon solved that problem by taking water aerobics. Exercise was suddenly fun! Marilyn found a real treasure in our local Fresh Fields Market with individual portions of both hot and cold dishes that fit right into her busy lifestyle. Food on the run no longer had to come from fast-food drive-throughs.

Marilyn worked her way up to cross-training five days a week for one hour. She admits it's still a challenge combining her new lifestyle changes and the activities of two growing boys, but this woman is up at dawn to get her exercise in. When her weight began to plateau she was discouraged (and who wouldn't be?). But when I explained to her and the class that a plateau simply means the body is making some adjustments, she looked at what she needed to adjust, too. After six months of the same exercise routine and a steady weight loss, it was time for Marilyn to increase the intensity level of her exercise and/or do different exercises and/or cut back on fat grams and calories. When another trainer gave her a free training session with new exercises that left her slightly sore, she started to see inches drop and eventually the scale drop as well. In order to keep Marilyn motivated I suggested that she stop weighing herself every day.

In October, 1999, Marilyn reached a milestone. She started out with her family on a beautiful bike trail in Monkton, Maryland, that would end in New Freedom, Pennsylvania, some twenty miles away. When the children started to slow down, Marilyn told her husband to stick with the children and said, "See ya later! I'm going to Pennsylvania!" Girlfriend made that trip with energy to spare!

Marilyn has lost seventy pounds and a total of fifty-four inches! Her goal is to lose thirty more pounds. I just know she's going to do it!

Plateaus and Weight Gain

Don't expect that just because you have made this new lifestyle change, you will lose weight every week without any problems. As you've seen with Marilyn (and myself), there will be weeks when your behavior toward food and exercise is excellent but you don't drop a pound. You may even gain a pound or two. Don't let this get you off-track and don't run to the nearest Dunkin' Donuts! I can't tell you how many times I hit plateaus and saw other members of my workshop do the same. I knew plateaus were a normal part of losing weight and could happen for any number of reasons—but hey, that doesn't mean I had to like them. What I didn't know, because I never stuck with any one diet for the long haul, was that the more weight you have to lose, the more plateaus you will hit before reaching your goal. Just as there are peaks and valleys in our daily life, so there are peaks and valleys in losing weight. The body needs to stop and get acquainted with its new status every once in a while. Our body makes many adjustments when losing weight. Once it has decided it's okay to have lost ten, twenty, or thirty pounds, then it will be ready to lose another ten, twenty, or thirty pounds. Plateaus can last for three or four weeks or even for a couple of months; it happened to me when I reached my halfway mark.

No one can eat or exercise perfectly all the time, nor should they. It's just not normal. In fact, I don't even like to use the word "perfect." Let's try *excellent* instead. Just remember this: Your body remembers everything you do because the cells in your body have memory. If you are eating and exercising properly, your body will activate that memory and you will move off the plateau. By the same measure, if you are not eating and/or exercising properly, your body will record every misstep on the scale and in the waistband of your favorite jeans! If you hit a plateau, ask yourself a few questions. What type of exercise am I doing? Am I weight training and building muscle? Or do I need something more aerobic? Am I writing in my journal? Am I drinking enough water?

While I was in basic/boot-camp training, we were doing tons of calisthenics and a lot of jogging. Since I'm a naturally muscular woman and tend to carry most of my weight in my thighs and buttock, I was starting to bulk up. My jeans were tighter around my thigh and buttock, area, but I still felt toned. The scale showed a weight gain, but I had lost inches in my waist. When basic training ended I talked to a few of the men and women and began to compare notes. Most of the naturally muscular men and women said they had gained weight *but* had lost inches. The men and women who tended to carry less weight from the waist down had either no weight gain or a small weight loss. Now I know how to adjust my exercise for different parts of my body.

And of course there is water retention. We, as women, are probably experts on water retention, since most of us deal with it at least once a month. Ladies, don't worry. You keep moving ahead and know that this is just temporary. Drink your water, eat plenty of natural diuretics like broccoli, asparagus, and watermelon, and relax. Speaking of relaxing, I also tend to retain water when I'm stressed. What about you? Have you noticed that certain foods or behaviors contribute to what I call the fat-finger syndrome?

November 5, 1995

> My weight has plateaued at 178 pounds. I know I can't get upset over this because it's only temporary. I have to keep telling myself that the scale should not be my only measure of weight loss. It should be my behavior toward exercise and food and how my clothes are fitting. I'm putting the scale away out of sight so I won't weigh myself every day. Out of sight, out of mind! My goal is to be healthy, not thin!

"Permanent" Plateau

After I lost 139 pounds, I couldn't seem to lose any more weight, no matter how excellent my eating and exercising. My body's memory bank seemed to be on vacation for an extended period of time. When I finally spoke to an expert about this, he explained that my weight had reached a permanent plateau. My body was so comfortable and so used to what I was feeding it and how I was exercising that if I wanted to lose more weight I either had to modify my eating, exercise with more intensity, or do both. That meant I either had to cut my food portions and/or fat intake and/or exercise at a higher intensity level. Now you know I was not tryin' to hear *nothin'* about eating less food because I knew I would feel deprived and start that vicious dieting cycle again. So I stepped up the intensity of my exercise routine and began to lose weight again. Ladies, increasing the intensity of your exercise means no longer strolling when you walk, especially if you have been at it for six months or more. It means strengthening the tension on your exercise bike or picking up a heavier weight. It means making another change. Step up the pace, drink more water, and let your face and body sweat to their heart's content. Don't worry about makeup; your face will be shiny with health! Even if I hadn't wanted to lose more weight, it was good to challenge myself and move to another level of excellence.

Stress or Illness

One winter I was bedridden and sick with the flu. I thought for sure that I would lose weight after not being able to eat anything for a few days. But when I weighed myself, I was not a happy woman. I had not only *not* lost weight, I had gained weight! But when I started to think logically about why I had gained weight, I remembered something very important. If you give your body too few calories, your metabolism literally slows down and actually prevents the loss of fat while breaking down muscle tissue. Your body begins to go into starvation mode, which is nothing more than a natural reaction to keep you alive. Your body is a very sophisticated engine and to operate properly, it needs fuel. (Remember this the next time you even think about going on a starvation diet.) Take advantage! Eat, eat, eat the right foods, exercise, write in your journal, and you will lose weight.

Occasional U-turns—Lapses and Relapses

As you know, sometimes keeping the weight off is harder than losing those unwanted pounds. After I lost my 157 pounds, I never for one minute thought I had licked my weight problem or that I was no longer a compulsive eater. I knew the greater challenge was still ahead—sticking to my lifestyle change for the rest of my life. Just like with all learning, I had to develop a set of skills and behaviors, and I had to practice them every day.

Did you ever take typing lessons? Remember having to practice the finger/letter positions without looking at the keyboard? Occasionally you would hit the *w* instead of the *q* or the *a* instead of the *s*. This new lifestyle isn't much different. You have to practice every day and some days you will hit the wrong key—*but what you do next makes all the difference.*

I had to prepare myself for the inevitable—occasional U-turns—lapses and relapses. I had to learn the difference between lapses and relapses and how they manifested themselves in my life. It's important to know the difference between the two because what you think about your eating makes a big difference in how you behave.

LAPSE: A temporary and minor slip. Just like a baby learning to walk will fall down at some points in its learning stages, you should be prepared to do the same. You *will* make some mistakes after losing all of your weight. I've had a lapse from time to time, but I know this is temporary and I will STOP it before it gets out of hand. Sometimes I gain weight, sometimes not. The more important issue is why. If I have a lapse more than once every two weeks, I know something is wrong. I'll make myself go back to writing a detailed food journal and spend extra time writing about what is eating me. Once I have identified the trigger food/behavior/ emotion, then I can set a plan of action for the next time.

One particular time I really overate after going to the gym. I had not eaten since 2:30 P.M., when I ate the last piece of fruit in my WAR bag (which you'll read about in the next chapter). By the time I arrived at the gym at 6 P.M., I was a little hungry, but by the time I finished my hour-long workout, I was starving! (I usually like to eat six small meals throughout the day.) I find when I stick to my usual workout time of 5:30 A.M., my hour-long workout does just the opposite and suppresses my appetite. But not that evening. I left the gym, jumped in my car and took off for the grocery store, taking the corners on two wheels. Don't ever get in the way of this hungry woman! Of course I bought everything in sight and ended up eating most of it before I even got home. Lesson learned? Now before going to the gym, I either eat a few hours before working out or pack enough fruit to eat immediately after my workout.

After a lapse it's important to:

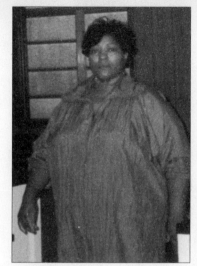

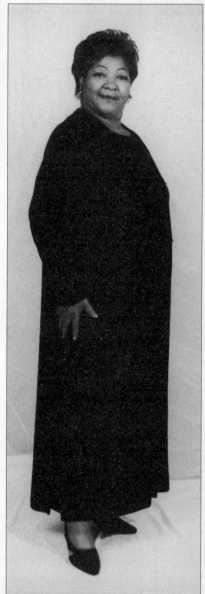

Vernell Ingram
Age: 56
Children: three sons (aged 30, 33, 39), one daughter (aged 31)
Grandchildren: 4
Starting weight: 258 pounds
Height: 5'3"
Weight lost to date: 40 pounds
Inches lost: 28

Photo by H. Alan Leo

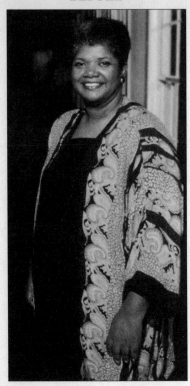

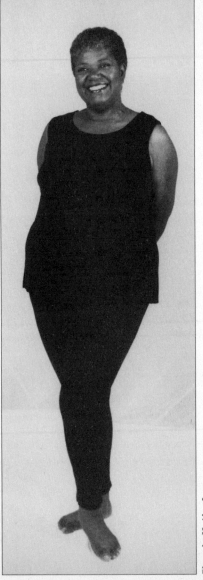

Vira Philips
Age: 62
Children: two sons (aged 42
    and one deceased at 33),
    two daughters (aged 40
    and 31), and adopted four
    children from the same
    family, two sons (aged 14
    and 15) and two daughters
    (aged 16 and one deceased
    at 16)
Grandchildren: 1
Starting weight: 252 pounds
Height: 5'5"
Weight lost to date: 20 pounds
Inches lost: 12

Photo by H. Alan Leo

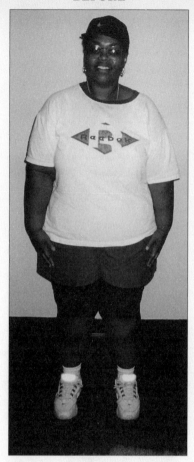

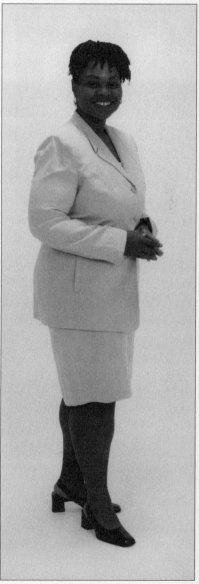

Marilyn McCraven
Age: 44
Children: two sons
    (aged 9 and 12)
Starting weight: 278 pounds
Height: 5'3"
Weight lost to date: 70 pounds
Inches lost: 30

Photo by H. Alan Leo

BEFORE

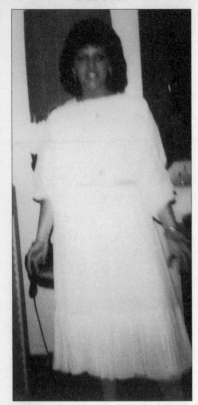

AFTER

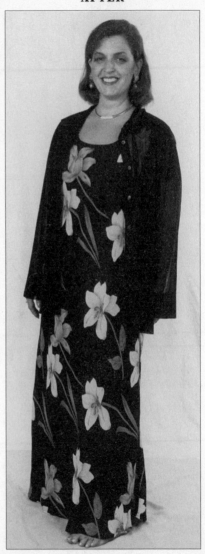

Phyllis G.
Age: 32
Single
Children: None
Starting weight: 208 pounds
Height: 5'3"
Weight lost to date: 50 pounds
Inches lost: 20

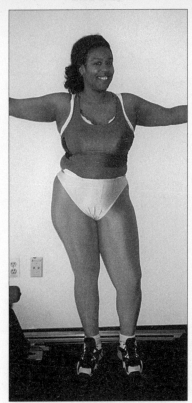

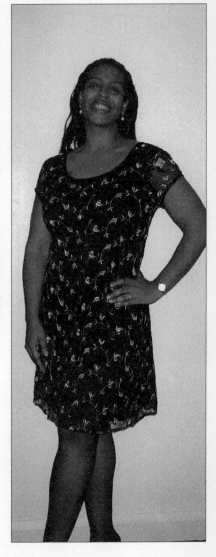

Jacquelyn Peterson
Age: 37
Married
Children: one son (aged 3),
  two daughters
  (aged 6 and 10)
Starting weight: 214 pounds
Height: 5'5"
Weight lost to date: 55 pounds
Inches lost: 41

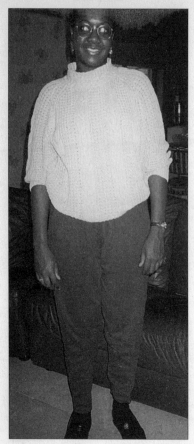

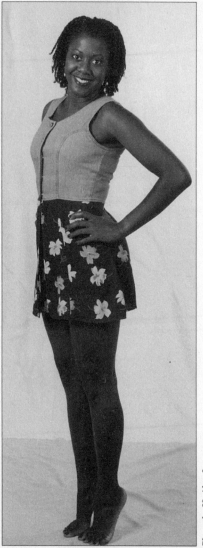

Kelley Phillips
Age: 31
Single
Starting weight: 160 pounds
Height: 5'6"
Weight lost to date: 30 pounds
Inches lost: 19

Photo by H. Alan Leo

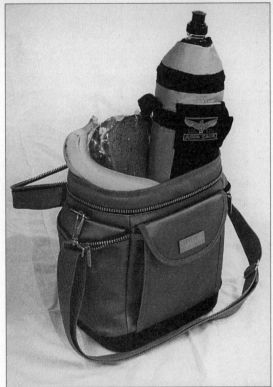

My WAR bag goes with me when I'm running errands on Saturdays.

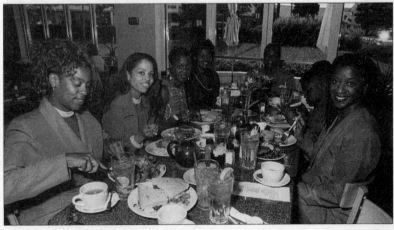

Having lunch at Donna's Cafe in Biblelot's bookstore. Celebrating with the ladies from the Through Thick & Thin Workshop™ after one of our photo shoots.

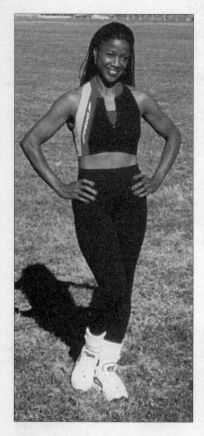

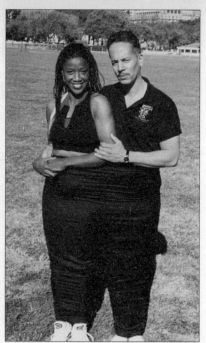

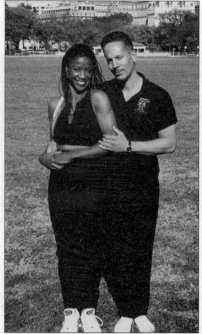

Ebony magazine photo shoot (January, 1998 issue). I'm standing in my old size 24 pants with Carroll.

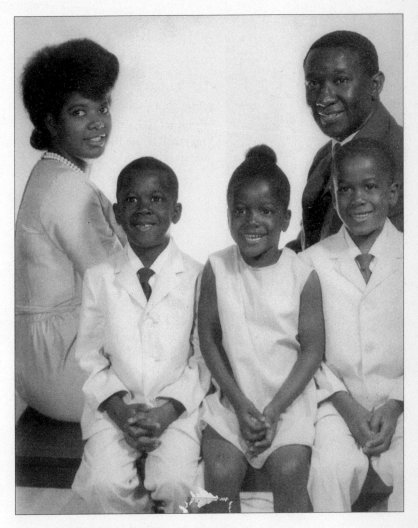

The Phillips family in 1965.
From left: Mom, Kevin, Crystal, Roy, Jr., and Dad.

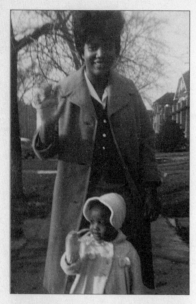

Mom and I hanging out, about to take our morning stroll while the boys are in school.

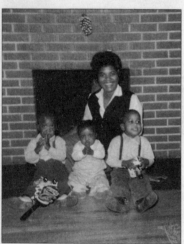

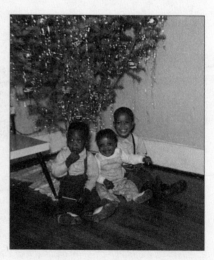

Here are the three of us celebrating Christmas. I am happy and smiling at the tender age of six months. Kevin is the one with the finger in his mouth. Roy, Jr. is to my right and was the ringleader, always getting us into trouble.

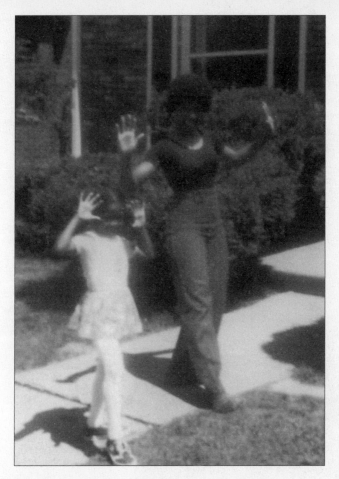

Kelley and I posing before I go to the dance studio. I'm a twelve-year-old girl living in a woman's body and hating every minute of my life at that time.

I deserve an Oscar for
the smiling performance
I put on at my wedding.
This was the most
unhappy day of my life.

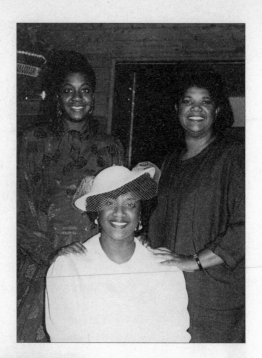

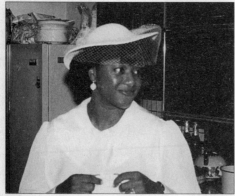

I wasn't crying tears of
joy at my wedding, I
cried because I knew I
was making a terrible
mistake.

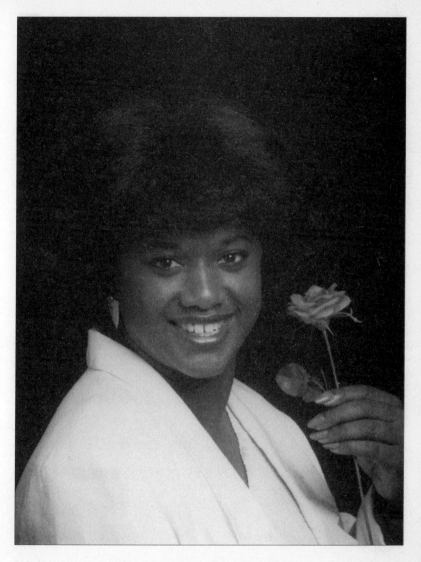

I did not want to take this picture because I felt like a cow holding this fake rose. I changed clothes six times before I found something that fit.

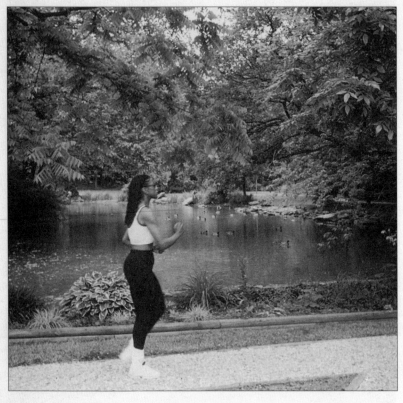

Me, power walking in one of the many peaceful and beautiful areas that I love to go to on nice summer days.

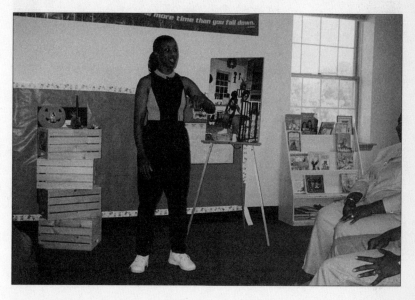

Presenting at a workshop to prepare the ladies for the kick-off of the holiday season—Halloween.

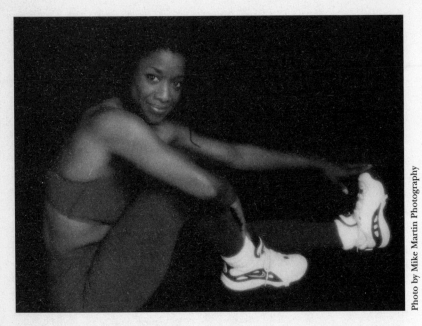

Me, finally at peace.

1. Know that nobody is perfect and you *will* occasionally overeat.
2. Accept the mistake for what it is—and move on (forgive yourself).
3. Stop and learn from your lapse. This is your chance to learn something new about behaviors you may need to change.
4. If you are part of a group like my workshop, Through Thick & Thin™, this is the perfect time to discuss your problems with the group or group leader.
5. Stop. Never say, "I've blown it now, so I may as well eat the rest of this and start again tomorrow." Remember, this is not a diet, this is a lifestyle change. Change the bad habit NOW!
6. Strive for excellence, not perfection.

RELAPSE: A relapse is a return, over an extended period of time, to your old eating behaviors. You have regressed and don't know whether you will recover. Just because you've had a relapse doesn't mean you have to stay there. I know you have fallen, but you *can* get up! When a child falls, do you encourage him or her just to lie there and never try to walk again? No, of course not, and neither should you.

Prepare for High-Risk Situations and Appropriate and Inappropriate Eating

Be careful of the three most common types of automatic thoughts that can lead you into high-risk situations: all-or-none thinking, doomsaying, and finding failure. After losing all my weight I said I would *never* eat ice cream or Popeye's chicken again. NOT. Not only is this not realistic but it makes certain foods illegal, and I don't want to label foods as good or bad. So instead of saying, "I'll never eat ice cream or Popeye's chicken again," I've set realistic and flexible goals like: "I can still eat ice cream or Popeye's chicken as long as I watch my calories and fat/sodium/carbohy-drate intake for the day. I can buy a Haagen-Dazs ice cream bar instead of a whole pint of ice cream. I can buy one or two pieces of fried chicken instead of an entire meal. I can find pleasure and sat-isfaction in moderation." Take care with how you position yourself and your relationship with food. Don't set yourself up by saying *never* or *when* or *bad*, or, perhaps worst of all, *it doesn't matter*.

Let me tell you about one of my most challenging experiences. I had out-of-town guests who drove in from Atlanta. I was scheduled to go out of town on business before they were to leave, so before I left I told them where the nearest grocery stores were just in case they ran out of something like coffee or toilet paper. Now, granted, I should have known that these dear Southern relatives of mine would not be interested in my nonfat yogurt, turkey salad, or tofu. After they left and I returned home late that same evening, I unpacked and went to the kitchen for something to eat. I opened the refrigerator and the freezer and, Lord have mercy, all of my old favorite binge foods were staring me right in the face! Homemade peach cobbler, leftover steak, a half gallon of gourmet ice cream, and half a slab of Uncle June Bug's famous barbecued ribs. I know they meant me no harm because this is the way my family has eaten for generations, but still, all my red flags were waving in the wind. What would you have done? What do you think I did?

1. — Put on the biggest muumuu I could find and start bingeing?
2. — Called all my friends over and had a party with the left-overs?
3. — Threw the leftovers in the trash?
4. — Ate a small helping of *some* of the leftovers and gave the rest away?
5. — Called my relatives and told them they needed to stop eating like this because it's unhealthy?
6. — Fed it to the dog?

7. —Paced back and forth, sweating and praying the left-overs would spoil by morning and went to bed dreaming about eating all night?
8. —Called 911 to report there was a lethal time bomb about to go off in my refrigerator?

If you guessed "Ate a small helping of *some* of the leftovers and gave the rest away," you read me like a book. I couldn't resist Uncle June Bug's ribs, so I ate two bones and had a spoonful of my favorite gourmet ice cream (Haagen-Dazs). Then I wrapped up the rest and took the leftovers to my neighbor, who has a big family to feed. I have to admit I did get an upset stomach later on that night. I think it was because I wasn't used to eating much pork, or maybe it was just a little too much fat for me in one sitting late at night. I was just thankful I didn't eat *everything* that night—I had "been there, done that" already and knew my old behavior would do nothing but lead me back to 292 pounds. I had truly embraced my new lifestyle change!

I've come up with the following early, middle, and late warning signs of relapse. I hope they will help you. Do they sound familiar? Have you "been there, done that"?

EARLY WARNING SIGNS
1. Thinking about certain food or food groups over and over again.
2. Craving certain foods or food groups.
3. Going places that serve your favorite food, but not going in.
4. Feeling uncomfortable when you are not overeating or bingeing.
5. Becoming resentful about having to work at keeping the weight off.
6. Believing that you are now over your problem as a compulsive eater and that you no longer have a weight problem.

7. Becoming anxious and fearful about the thought of eating certain foods.

8. Becoming restrictive about what you eat, believing any deviance from your eating plan will cause you to overeat or binge.

9. Avoiding parties, banquets, ceremonies, or any occasion where food will be front and center.

10. Avoiding people who like to eat or eat out in restaurants.

11. Wanting to return to a restricted regime like fasting, food supplements, or diet pills.

12. Worrying extensively about regaining your weight.

MIDDLE WARNING SIGNS

13. Having frequent discussions about your eating habits or someone else's.

14. Moderately starting to eat certain food groups that you used to binge on.

15. Beginning to put on weight but telling yourself you will take it off later.

16. Having an "I don't care" attitude about your weight.

17. Thinking constantly about your weight, eating habits, and body shape.

18. Becoming angry with others when they say anything about your food or weight.

19. Starting to worry about everything but you and putting your exercise and journal writing on the back burner.

20. Eating at irregular times.

21. Having difficulty managing stress without overeating.

22. Having problems falling asleep or going to sleep without eating something.

23. Sleeping more than normal or exercising sporadically.

LATE WARNING SIGNS

24. Overeating to manage tense, negative feelings such as anger, sadness, or anxiety.
25. Having feelings of self-pity that life is so difficult because of your weight problem.
26. Using medications or drugs/alcohol to deal with stress.
27. Losing your self-confidence to manage overeating episodes.
28. Lying to yourself and others about what you eat, how much you eat, and what your weight is now.
29. Having problems managing work, family, and friends without overeating or eating compulsively.
30. Feeling powerless, hopeless, and helpless about managing your weight and starting to binge.
31. Thinking seriously of having an operation like lyposuction to change how your body looks.
32. Playing out fantasies of suicide.

One of my favorite sayings is "A Bend in the Road Is Not the End of the Road . . . Unless You Fail to Make the Turn." The road will not end if you lapse or relapse. The tools are still there. Your basic foundation is still in place. You know what works and what doesn't. You know how glorious a good food day can be. And, remember you are not alone.

10

THIS IS WAR!
(WRITE, AWARE, REASONABLE)

*I*t's a WAR out there when it comes to eating right—especially when your goal is to stop dieting and commit to a lifestyle change. Does your lifestyle keep you so busy you think you can't possibly find the time to fit exercise or journal writing into your schedule? Is preparing a bag lunch out of the question because it's easier and takes less time to grab something on the run? Well, all those things may be true, but if you really want to lose that weight, then you have some decisions to make. I promise you, my schedule was about as full as you can imagine. But when I finally decided I was the most important person in my life, a few magic time slots opened. This really is about priorities. Is it more important to spend an extra thirty minutes in bed in the morning or to lose weight? Is it more important to get carry-out for lunch, or really to live your life? Is it more important to watch that stupid TV game show or spend thirty minutes walking your way to happiness? You have children and a husband? Congratulations—but don't think for one minute that makes you exempt. Some of my best clients are proud, lookin'-good mamas!

This is what my life looked like—keeping abreast of the ever-changing pharmaceutical industry, working ten-hour days, entertaining customers on the weekends and in the evenings so I could get in to see them the next week, working late into the night to finish paperwork for the home office, and all the while trying to stay in the top one-third for sales numbers. I wanted a better life for myself and seriously started to climb the corporate ladder. I began accepting special projects like training local representatives and then traveling to New Jersey to assist the national trainer. The advent of managed care changed everything I knew about selling and I was faced with changing or leaving the industry. I was no longer a fairly normal-sized energetic college graduate. I was tired and fat and felt a hundred years old. I had finally managed to show most of my important doctor clients that just because I was fat, African-American, and female, it didn't mean I was stupid. Now I had to learn a whole new way of selling. The evolution of managed care was supposed to offer structure, but instead it was starting to ruin my body and the structured box I had built around me. How was I going to find time to exercise, write in my journal, eat a balanced meal in peace, brush up on new selling techniques, or even walk Heru? I had to decide how to streamline my overflowing plate in order to streamline my waistline and save myself from the streamlining that was starting to occur in the pharmaceutical industry. I had to find balance and prioritize what was important in my life. In fact, I had to create a whole new way of living and being.

In this chapter I'll share with you how my WAR bag saw me through when I was busy, traveling, stressed, bored, pissed off, or deliriously happy when I managed to get quality time with a difficult-to-see doctor. I'll also show you a plan of action that will help you deal with smart, on-the-run food shopping, eating at the fast-food drive-through, and grabbing a snack from the shelves of a

convenience store. It's a food war out there, and you have to protect that good foundation you have been building for yourself.

I'm not gonna lie and tell you it was easy for me to stop the bad
habit of grabbing something quick and unhealthy to eat on the
run. It's tough breaking old habits even when you know they're
not good for you. I learned to use Sunday as a staging ground for
the rest of the week. Pretty early on in this process I realized that if
I had food with me at all times, then I could eat whenever I was
hungry. That was important to me. Just as I wanted food that tasted
good, I also wanted to be able to eat on my schedule, not someone else's. (Besides, what if I totally lost it and binged my way
through my WAR bag? At least I would be bingeing on healthy
food!)

After I came in from church on Sunday I would head for the
kitchen. I'd prepare a few days' worth of meals and snacks and put
them away in the refrigerator, all ready to pop into my bag. My
WAR bag is a lightweight, weatherproof safety net armed with fuel
that feeds my stomach and nourishes my soul. I call it WAR bag
because it helps me to stay honest by WRITING daily in my journal
and being AWARE enough to make REASONABLE choices. First, I start
with my 10 A.M. snack—a banana or half a bagel with just a slide of
butter or margarine. Lunch was usually around 1:30 P.M. and I
would take thirty to forty-five minutes with NO distractions. No cell
phone, no radio, no newspaper. I wanted to focus on every morsel
I put into my mouth. Why not? I was eating stir-fried greens, crispy
catfish, and a piece of buttermilk cornbread. Add sixteen ounces
of distilled water, and I was set until about 4 P.M. Then it was time
for what I think is the perfect fruit—cool, sweet, sliced mango. But
that wasn't the last of my food. I always tucked in what I called my
"mad" food—maybe a one-ounce bag of potato chips or pretzels.
(Yes, I said potato chips, but please check out the serving size.) I
didn't always use it but I knew if I got angry or upset, my mouth
would start calling for something crunchy. There's just something
about biting down hard that is so satisfying. If I'm working a par-

ticularly challenging part of my territory, then I'll pack two chopped carrots and a cucumber—my teeth need to work more when I'm fussing in the car about a difficult doctor.

My WAR bag goes with me packed and ready if I'm gone for more than two hours. I also pack my WAR bag, especially for my sweet tooth, when I am going out of town. Plane, train, or car, it doesn't matter. And I always keep ready food at my apartment. Sometimes, when I'm riding my stationary bike, commercials for Popeye's come on and I find myself drooling more than sweating. Then I need to be sidetracked from running right out that door and down the street.

The last thing you would ever see Crystal Jayne with when she weighed 292 pounds was a packed lunch from home. Even when I used to go to the salon to have my hair permed, knowing I would have to wait a while for my appointment, I *never* took anything to eat. I would have died first before allowing anyone to see me eat something in public. Breaking out of that binge mind-set—squirreling away food, hiding it, and eating large quantities when it was safe—was something I thought I'd never be able to overcome. I still have my moments, but nothing like the old days. I had to overcome that small inner voice that said, "How will it look for a 292-pound woman to carry around a packed lunch? You know everybody will be thinking, 'The last thing she needs to do is eat!' " I also had to challenge myself to grow a backbone, especially when my hair stylist was running forty minutes behind schedule. Like a fool I still wouldn't go out to get something to eat or tell her I would no longer need her services. Instead I would sit and wait, getting increasingly nauseated and light-headed. And, girl, I was starving! The truth is I didn't want to have to struggle in front of everyone getting up from the soft-cushioned sofa or have everyone watch my huge thighs and behind waddle next door to the Chinese carry-out. As a result, half my day was spent in the hair salon feeling weak and miserable. When I finally left, burning scalp and all, I'd drive like a crazy woman, not to the nearest emergency room, but to the nearest drive-through window. But that was yesterday. Today I have my WAR bag

There are a few days when I forget to take my WAR bag, or Sunday is so busy I don't have time to cook those good whole meals. On those days I will pick up something from a fast-food drive-through or go in to eat if I can spare twenty minutes. The difference now is in what I order. If I'm running late, I'll go to a Wendy's and get a grilled chicken sandwich without the sauce and a garden salad. Sometimes I'm in the mood for pizza, so I'll go to Pizza Hut and order two slices from a 10-inch (small pizza) thin and crispy cheese pizza, which is low in fat (just five grams for one slice), and a salad.

If I'm mall shopping without my WAR bag, I head straight to Chick-Fil-A. They, by far, have the tastiest and lowest-in-fat chicken around. They even have the calorie and fat-gram information on their bag, comparing it to the competition. This is the only place I know of that I can get my groove on with chicken nuggets that aren't high as the sky in fat grams. An eight-piece Chick-Fil-A chicken nugget is fourteen grams of fat and 290 calories, compared to McDonald's nine-piece Chicken McNuggets' twenty-six grams of fat and 430 calories. Chick-Fil-A's char-grilled chicken deluxe sandwich with lettuce and tomato is only three grams of fat. Since the meals are so low in fat and calories, I add a small salad, and every blue moon, if I've banked my fat grams, I'll have a slice of their lemon pie for desert. Subway also has a great selection of low-fat sandwiches, just look for their lite menu.

You must know by know I can't live without my occasional Popeye's for long. Now I order a one-piece, okay, so sometimes it's a two-piece meal. But I only order white meat and I only order the chicken. Those biscuits have as many grams of fat as one chicken breast. If I run into a convenience store, I have to be careful because the doughnuts and pizzas are *loaded* with fat. The rotating hot dogs aren't much better, so the safest item for me to purchase is a small bag of pretzels and a small bottle of juice or a large bottled water. The only convenience store where I'll grab real food is a local neighborhood health food store.

You can eat on the run, if you have to. You just have to think it through and come up with a game plan.

On weekends when I want delicious, good-for-me food, I like to meet friends for lunch at "Donna's Café" in one of my local "Bibelot's" bookstores. Everything is wonderful, fresh, and prepared with love. My favorites are the Sicilian tuna sandwich on multi-grain bread with green and black olives, capers, pepperoncini, and greens, with a half order of "Donna's" famous roasted vegetable (eggplant, artichoke hearts, red peppers, onions, beets, cauliflower, carrots, and red and green peppers) salad. I also love the roasted turkey with provolone and spicy olive-pepper relish on a baguette. If I'm out on a date I like to steer us to "Houston's" for the consistently good grilled salmon or lake trout. Both places are reasonably priced and help me keep a reasonable waistline. "Mr. Chan's" in Pikesville fills my Chinese craving with a wonderful vegetarian menu.

For smart-on-the-run food shopping I'll run into our local grocery store with a list of two days' worth of quick convenience foods to buy. I don't always have time to cook a week's worth of meals on Sunday, so I'll purchase a lunch- or dinner-portion entrée from the frozen food section that is tasty and low in fat. If the rotisserie chicken is looking good and calling my name, I'll buy one along with a side dish of vegetables and take that for lunch or have it for dinner for a few days. Sometimes I'll go to the salad bar and fix myself a fresh salad—but I wait till I get home to add my salad dressing. If I want something sweet, I'll buy frozen low-fat yogurt or fresh fruits like peaches, nectarines, or mangoes.

Now let's take a look at how many calories and fat grams I save myself with smart shopping—on the run or planning ahead.

292 lbs. eating	135 lbs. eating

Breakfast

Sausage egg muffin
  29 fat grams, 440 calories
Chocolate-glazed doughnut
  24 fat grams, 410 calories
Total: 53 fat grams, 850 calories

Mango 0.5 fat grams,
135 calories

0.5 fat grams, 135 calories

Snack

99-cent bag of chips
  35 fat grams, 490 calories

TOTAL: 35 fat grams, 490 calories

Pretzels 1-oz., 1 fat gram,
  110 calories

1 fat gram, 110 calories

Lunch

Philly cheese steak sub
  47 fat grams, 755 calories

TOTAL: 47 fat grams, 755 calories

Roasted turkey sandwich
  12 fat grams, 385 calo-
  ries—Side salad 4 fat
  grams, 70 calories
16 fat grams, 455 calories

Snack

nothing

Peach no fat grams,
  45 calories

Dinner

Corned-beef sandwich
  6-oz. 50 fat grams,
  632 calories

TOTAL: 50 fat grams, 632 calories

Vegetarian lasagna 10
  fat grams,
  300 calories,
  side salad 4 fat grams,
  70 calories
14 fat grams, 370 calories

Dessert   Frozen low-fat yogurt

                                     (1 cup) 3 fat grams,

                                     240 calories

TOTALS

185 fat grams, 2,727 calories   34.5 fat grams, 1355 cal.

All fat-gram and calorie counts are from two sources: *The Completely Revised*
and Updated Fast-Food Guide, second edition; and *The Complete & Up-to-*
Date Fat Book.

Look at the difference in my body fat:

292-lbs   **135-lbs.**

body fat: 52.3%   22%

Lordy, lordy, I was sure to die before my time eating like that!
I've cut 150.5 fat grams out of my diet, reducing my daily fat grams
almost four times. I have also cut my calories almost in half and my
daily fat and calorie intake varies depending on how hard a workout I've had for the day.

My WAR bag is filled with nutritious foods that I know I can eat
for the rest of my life. It's not packed with diet foods that leave me
feeling deprived, angry, and hungry. When I packed my WAR bag
I made sure I packed it with foods that satisfied me mentally as
well as physically so I would feel no shame writing about my food
in my journal. I write about my snacks and lunch and whether or
not they prevented me from going to fast-food places to fill up on
cheap fuel. WRITING honestly made me keenly AWARE of my food
and how I used it. Writing also pushed me to make REASONABLE
choices about portion sizes. Initially I was self-conscious about my
WAR bag. People used to snicker when they saw my 250-pound self
carrying around an insulated bag. My neighbor used to look at my
huge lunch carrier and slowly shake her head. I wanted to tell her
I had quality whole foods in my lunch bag and knew what I was
doing. But I decided I'd let the results speak for me.

Days I craved fried lake trout were the days I took my crispy cat-fish. Fresh peaches and low-fat yogurt took the place of peach cob-bler. I could always find something to substitute, it just took a bit of thinking. The food I lovingly prepared made the foods I used to eat taste like junk! I stopped working through my lunch hour and started enjoying my quiet time. I ate with no distractions. I didn't read, listen to fast music, or talk on the phone. I wanted to be aware of every bite. I wanted really to taste and savor my food. Never again did I want to sit and wonder what happened to my food like I used to when I ate in a state of constant confusion and distraction.

The morning is my favorite part of the day. I love sitting in the quiet stillness perched in my window seat with a cup of something warm and satisfying. Just watching the birds and squirrels and an occasional deer helps me to appreciate that God has given me the strength and courage to see my way through and I thank him for another day.

Reeducating myself about food, listening to my body, keeping my health a priority, adding variety, and trusting my instincts—this is what helps me stay centered. Keeping excess baggage at a mini-mum makes my life flow with simplicity and balance. When I traveled as the district trainer from Pennsylvania to Maryland, Washington, D.C., Virginia, and North Carolina, I couldn't always pack a lunch. I kept my fast-food guide at my side and concen-trated on restaurants that grilled their food. I would also find the local health food stores if I wanted sweets without refined sugar. If the hotel didn't have a fitness center I wouldn't stay there. The fit-ness center also had to offer convenient hours that fit *my* schedule. Was I being selfish and self-centered? Was I putting me first? You bet!

Now, let's look at what I needed to learn about nutrition. Isn't it amazing that the average American's weight has increased every year for the past decade? Are we really eating more, or just making poorer choices? Personally, I wanted to learn everything I could about nutrition because to enjoy the process of losing weight I had to know how processed food affected my body. People who read my story and join my weight-loss workshop always want to know what I eat. It's not magic and I didn't have to go back to school to learn what I needed. First, I read everything I could get my hands on and then made some *intelligent* choices for the long haul and for my overall health. I could fuel my body with low-grade foods (add low fat, no fat to that list) and get slow, undependable results, or I could incorporate real high-grade food into my menus and get quality results. You you don't have to be a genius on this one.

My food pyramid used to look like this:

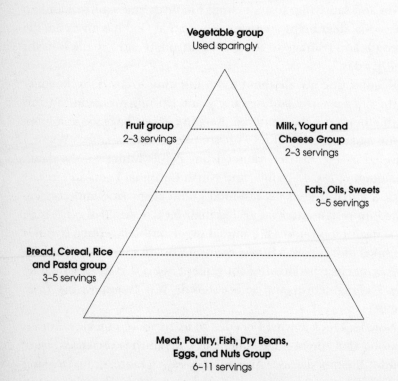

Vegetable group
Used sparingly

Fruit group
2–3 servings

Milk, Yogurt and Cheese Group
2–3 servings

Fats, Oils, Sweets
3–5 servings

Bread, Cereal, Rice and Pasta group
3–5 servings

Meat, Poultry, Fish, Dry Beans, Eggs, and Nuts Group
6–11 servings

I rarely ate whole fresh vegetables, and my fruit usually came from a can with heavy syrup to make peach cobblers. Refined breads and pastas with added fats and sugars were my staples, and nuts were always straight out of a jar or can and roasted with plenty of salt and added sugars. I cooked my eggs with butter and made grilled-cheese sandwiches with tons of bacon inside. I ate Haagen-Dazs ice cream by the pint and always bought meats with visible fats and then fried them. Saturated fats and hydrogenated oils were all I ever used. I sweetened my drinks, cereals, and deserts with white refined sugar or chemical sweeteners. I was the picture of death, a testimony to the saying, "You are what you eat."

When I talk to overweight people or yo-yo dieters, they all tell me the same thing. "I think something's wrong with my metabolism because in order to lose weight I have to eat one meal a day. Whenever I eat more than one meal I gain weight." Most of them reason that since they have a slow metabolism, they don't need much food and their fat will burn off with less food. NOT! We have been programmed to diet and conditioned to starve. Starving yourself will only lessen your ability to burn calories or fat. When you deny your body fuel, a red flag starts signaling your brain, warning that famine is just around the corner. (Remember the cultural heritage and what starving does to your body discussion in Chapter 5?)

As a survival instinct, your body slows its metabolic rate way below the level needed to maintain your weight. The body is in such a panic at the prospect of hunger that you may lose a few pounds initially, but after that the mind/body connection starts to shut down. Under these conditions your body is happy just to keep your weight at the same level, no more, no less. When you diet like this, you will not lose pounds proportionate to the number of calories you are consuming. The harder you push your body to lose weight, the more your body will work stubbornly against you.

In order for a fire to burn or a car to run, it needs fuel. In order for your body to lose, you have to fuel it and move it. My fuel turned out to be what I call whole foods. I felt better, looked better, and lost weight faster. The next time you make a trip to the grocery store, look into the fresh produce and fruit section. Try incorporating fresh vegetables and fruits into your new lifestyle at least a few days out of the week. I know canned foods last longer and are much easier to keep, but trust me on this. Your taste buds will thank you.

What are whole foods? When a food is in its natural form, whether rooted underground, hanging from a tree, or attached to a bush, it is a whole food. It has the most energy, the most life, and the most nutrients. Now I don't expect you to go dig, pick, or pull your own foods, but at least you will know what to look for. You want foods that have not been altered since leaving their source of origin. You want *fresh*. When I eat whole foods I notice my blood sugar levels stay steady, my craving for sugar subsides, and my body's elimination system works better. I'm simply happier and don't think about food every minute of the day. A nutrient-dense food gives me more satisfaction than any low-fat, no-fat food ever could. I used to think quantity would fill my stomach, but after a while I noticed that low-fat, no-fat, processed, and prepared foods left me feeling hungry and then I ate increased portions to make up for what I was missing. I was one of those people who got fat on low-fat, no-fat diets. These foods were usually made with highly processed sugar, flour, and chemical sweeteners. The foods had no life to them and they made my life not worth living.

What about lean foods versus fat foods? When I stopped dieting I had to stop viewing fat as bad and the only thing that counted in a diet to lose weight. In fact, our bodies need added fat. They just need to be the right fats. Looking at everything as a whole—fat, fiber, calories, and sugar—was an education in itself. At one point I thought I would become a vegetarian in order to lose weight, but quickly learned that vegetarians can be overweight too. Cheeses, nuts, seeds, and dairy products can all add up.

Just because something doesn't have meat or fat or sugar or dairy doesn't mean you can have all you want. Balance, moderation, symmetry, equilibrium—got the picture? I was fat because my whole life was an either/or situation. Now I look for that balance, moderation, symmetry, equilibrium in everything I do and eat. I don't eat much meat or dairy, and when I do I look for organic products. I've noticed that large amounts of hormones or antibiotics in red meat, chicken, and dairy products leave me bloated and reaching for a larger than normal bra. When I occasionally eat meat I eat lean meats with no hormones or antibiotics (free range). I eat plenty of fish now because it doesn't leave me feeling and looking bloated. Look for meat cuts that are lean. Marbled steak is not the good fat your body needs. Dark meat has more fat than light meat, but it also has more flavor. If that's your choice, just eat a smaller amount. Remember the type of meat you eat can contribute to excess fat.

Canola oil and olive oil (from plant sources) are much healthier than oils from animal sources. Both of these oils are better for you than cream, butter, or fatty meats, and they taste wonderful. Initially I was not a believer in using canola oil or olive oil because I thought it would compromise the taste of my food. I would have never believed that canola oil would taste just as good as fat-back in my collard greens but you must taste it yourself to believe it. In fact, I can taste my food better without all the animal fat. Because we aren't used to it, two tablespoons of oil may not seem like a lot but, trust me, the flavor from those two tablespoons is worth a cup of anything else.

Try Going Nude . . .
When you think of mashed potatoes, french fries, or rice, do you automatically think gravy? I know I used to. I'd get fightin' mad if I couldn't sop up my biscuit or roll with some gravy or heavy sauce. Yes, I still love gravy, but there are some other things that taste almost as good—like broth-based sauces and vinaigrettes. Your

heart has to work hard enough every day just propelling you around—don't make it any harder by clogging your arteries with globs of fat. Save your gravy days for Thanksgiving or Christmas and then enjoy them to the fullest. Make a healthy decision for today and move on.

Is Your Food Dead or Alive?

A "live" food is unaltered. It has not been stored or processed. If you plant a peach in the ground, you *could* get a peach tree in return. If you plant peaches from a can, the possibility of getting a peach tree is zero. Live foods like raw carrots, cucumbers, peppers, cauliflower, asparagus, pea pods, sprouts, raw peanuts, and even potatoes are exponentially better for our health than the same items fully cooked and canned or frozen. When foods are cooked we kill the enzymes our system needs to digest and utilize nutrients. Cooked foods, no matter how tasty, put a burden on our digestive system. As professional dieters we have all heard about rabbit food. Don't eat raw foods as a substitute for something you really want, don't eat raw foods to fill you up, and don't feel like you have to eat raw foods every day of the week. Do eat raw foods once, twice, maybe even three times a week because they can change the quality of your life and make losing those unwanted pounds a lot easier. Sounds like a no-brainer to me.

Listening to Your Body

Most babies and small children are naturally slim because they are in touch with their natural drives and instincts. They eat only when they are hungry and stop eating when they are satisfied. I had to become a child again and learn to listen to my body. I had to let go of the fear and trust the process. Instincts are not lost, they may be confined, subdued, or hidden, but they are with us until the day we die. Life experiences make us question our natural instincts, and the less we get involved in taking care of ourselves in mind, body, and spirit, the less in tune we are with our natural instincts. I had to learn to stop automatically eating at noon just because it was noon or because someone else wanted to or because someone had fixed something for me. My internal clock likes to dine later in the day.

I have also become a picky eater. Me, who used to eat almost everything in sight. I love myself now and I care about what foods I choose to fuel my body. When I want to eat I stop to think, "Am I really hungry or am I using food to comfort myself emotionally or spiritually?" For a long time this was all I knew. Now that I know better, I'm doing better. Sometimes after eating I find myself looking for something else to eat knowing that I'm not physically hungry. So I check myself for nutrient hunger. Was it a balanced meal? Did I eat any fresh fruits or vegetables? With all the fast food and microwaves around, it's easy to go for days without fresh foods. Balance in eating, exercising, resting, and learning are difficult for me. Eliminating words like *never, always, perfection,* and *obsession* have allowed me to stop living an all-or-nothing life. I'm constantly moving to the right, left, forward, and sometimes backward. But I'm always striving to move closer and closer to the center.

Variety Is the Spice
Eating the same foods over and over bores me to tears. I found that adding a variety of tastes to my meals helped me to lose weight, but it also offered me better nutrition. Try different textures as well as tastes, colors, and temperatures. Hot, cold, liquid, solid, smooth, chewy, crunchy, thin, thick, red, white, purple, green. Food is meant to be enjoyed as much as it is meant to be fuel.

My Health Is My Priority
If you don't have your health, you have nothing. Ever wonder why this saying has been around as long as you can remember? Because it's true! You can have all the riches in the world but if you are not well you won't have the energy to enjoy them. My goal was not just to get rid of my fat body, but to attend to my health and my life. My goal was to find balance, and that process is ongo-

ing. Staying healthy mentally, physically, and spiritually allows me to wake up before dawn to enjoy the sounds of nature. Staying healthy allows me to travel and see the sun rise in a different part of the world. Feeling healthy and being healthy makes me happy—not being in a smaller dress size. I've lost weight before, thinking that it would make me happy, but it didn't work. Learning to love myself tastes better than any food in the world.

Changing me inside is what really made the difference in my outside appearance and the way I live my life. It's not about changing just one thing—it's about the whole enchilada! You will only get back what you give in return. If you continue to eat fast foods on the run and don't exercise on a regular basis, you will get limited results. When you start taking time to incorporate exercise and healthy foods into your lifestyle, you'll get the results you want—and want to keep for a lifetime.

It's a food war out there! Fill your WAR bag, prepare yourself for battle, and seize the day! It's yours for the taking.

Here are two special ladies from my workshop who have learned to incorporate change and their WAR bag into their hectic lives.

Phyllis G.

Age 32—single
Children: none
Starting weight: 208 lbs.
Height: 5'3"
Weight lost to date: 50 lbs.
Inches lost: 20

Life was tough for Phyllis growing up in New York City. Walking down the busy streets of Manhattan was pretty depressing for her when she constantly saw beautiful women who looked like models or actresses brushing past her. She used to subscribe to all the fashion magazines and daydream about being thin and gorgeous like the women on the pages. There's a saying that most still hold to: "You can never be too thin or too rich." Phyllis had to learn the too-thin part the hard way.

She was known as "Fat Phyllis" in her neighborhood. When she was twelve years old, she weighed 190 pounds and hadn't even reached her adult height of five feet three. Phyllis always felt miserable and bloated. Her dieting career started around that time, when her mother took her to the doctor. Phyllis was prescribed the same diet pills that her mother was on to lose weight. The side effects were horrible. She couldn't sleep, her heart raced, and she was jumpy all the time. When she stopped taking the diet pills, the weight came back on, so she put herself on a six-hundred-calorie diet. By the end of the first week, Phyllis was so hungry she started bingeing. Afterward, she feared she would gain all the weight back and started purging. Phyllis would go for long periods of time without eating. She suffered with anorexia nervosa and bulimia for fifteen years. Her weight ranged from 208 pounds to 132 pounds, as Phyllis was always losing and gaining it back rapidly. She suffered from the disease to please and found it hard to say no to people or to defend herself when someone attacked her with vicious words. As a result, she always put herself down and felt that she was not thin enough or pretty enough when relationships failed. At an early age Phyllis watched her parents' marriage slowly dissolve. She saw her mother struggle to make ends meet for her and her sister after her father left.

Phyllis's eating disorder became out of control and she was hospitalized after she blacked out from not eating for days. During and after the hospital stay, she gained fifty pounds in two months. Finally she sought professional help and has not gone back to any of the eating disorders. But Phyllis was left with the extra weight and has stayed at the same weight for four years. This is a great accomplishment for her in one sense because her weight never stayed the same for more than a few days when she was anorexic/bulimic, but now she is looking for a healthy weight as well as a healthy way to reduce.

Phyllis works as a speech pathologist. Like me, she travels in her car for hours going to various locations. Usually she does not eat breakfast. Around 10 A.M. while driving, she'll get hungry and stop off at a convenience store to grab a candy bar or a sandwich. By 4 P.M. she is very sluggish and tired and wants to go home to eat. Sometimes Phyllis would make any excuse to leave work to get home to eat. The next day she would call in sick because she ate too much the night before and felt sick and disgusted. While taking off for a sick day she justified it by saying, "I need this day to get myself together so I can be my best and start off on the right track for tomorrow." Of course by the time 10 A.M. rolled around, she went to the store again for her sugar fix and would crash once more by 4 P.M.

One day while driving to work she heard my story on radio 92-Q in Baltimore. She was moved by my years of struggling to lose weight. Phyllis wrote down the phone number of my weight-loss workshops. That evening she drove from western Maryland, which is three hours away, in record time to attend my workshop.

Initially, Phyllis's progress was slow because she was too busy thinking what she needed to do instead of just doing it. When she finally started doing the work, her weight started melting away. What's different about her weight loss this time is that she's not angry, because she has stopped dieting. I admire Phyllis for not being afraid to eat whatever she wants in moderation and not labeling foods as good or bad. For the first time in a long time, she can see and feel her collarbone. A few weeks ago when she went shopping, she tried on a size 16 and it was too big. At first she thought it must be a big size 16 so she tried on other size 16s and they were all too big. When she tried on a size 12, it fit just right! Phyllis went to New York the following week to see her mother, and when they went shopping she tried on a size 16 again, thinking still that the clothes in that other store must have had big size

16s that day. Phyllis's mother told her to take off the size 16 when she came out of the dressing room to show her the dress. Her mother said it was too big!

Today Phyllis is truly a size 10. While the photographer was taking her after picture, I wanted to scream and shout for joy because she looked so beautiful. I also had to tell Phyllis to stop wearing size 12 clothes because they were hanging off her little body. I have seen an amazing transformation not only in Phyllis's weight but also in her spirit. This woman has now learned to say no and has learned to tell guys to take a hike when they think she's not thin enough to be the trophy bimbo on their arm.

I'm so proud of Phyllis because she made time out of her busy schedule to attend *every* workshop. She has not only managed to control her eating disorder, she has managed to love herself again!

Jacquelyn Peterson

Age: 37—married
Mother of one son (3 years) and two daughters (6 and 10 years)
Starting weight: 214 lbs.
Height: 5'5"
Weight lost to date: 55 lbs.
Inches lost: 41

Jacquelyn often had sluggish feelings, recurring asthma attacks, and noticeable changes in the structure of her teeth. She thought the additional hair strands in the brush and the obvious weight gain were just the result of being in her middle thirties, having had three children, and living a congested life. She ignored that internal voice that kept whispering, "Pay attention to me. I need your help. I'm not supposed to feel like this." Her response was always the same—"Ignore it! I'm too busy to listen." A typical superwoman's response.

Jacquelyn's awakening point was in December 1997. She and

her best friend were having a much-needed girls' night out. They were excited. They purchased similar dresses, went to the hairdresser, and put on makeup. They posed proudly for their photo. A week later Jacquelyn received the photo back. The results were devastating! She was ashamed and saddened at how her once size 12 frame had ballooned to a size 18/20. She recognized that her overall health was out of control and that she had to listen to the voice within and respond.

Jacquelyn's main obstacle was how to break the superwoman cycle and concentrate on herself. Everything seemed to be important: laundry, meals, homework, housework. Make time for exercise and proper nutrition? When? How?

On a local radio station Jacquelyn heard me addressing some of these issues. Jacquelyn came to my workshop with her three beautiful children and her supportive husband, who handles the hardware—Gregory is a computer whiz! I was elated that she was determined not to pass her old lifestyle on to her children. She wanted to break old eating habits that were passed down to her.

To improve her body, she joined a local gym. To improve her mind, she stuck with the group workshop. Her physical routine began with simple strength building and agility tasks. Jacquelyn also had a great desire to increase her endurance and aspire to new goals, but she was vulnerable to doubts and fear. Hindering thoughts slowed her down. "What if I've gone too far with the weight gain and I fail at losing weight? How long does it take before anyone notices any results?" Being a member of the workshop allowed her to voice her fears and encouraged her to pass through the fear while maintaining her passion for progress. I helped to relieve her worries by reassuring her that she had the right attitude and could soar at great altitudes. I also reminded her that challenges are not supposed to be easy and that quitting is always an option, but is not the solution to healing the body.

By early spring of 1998, Jacquelyn had found a great exercise partner. The two began to walk in just about every walk-a-thon Baltimore had to offer. They shared fitness facts and nutritional assessments. By the fall of 1998, Jacquelyn had braces on her teeth, braids in her hair, and a weight loss of twenty pounds. Today Jacquelyn has not only managed to lose fifty-five pounds and forty-one inches, she was also featured in a major fitness magazine that shared her success with the world. Her energy level is up and her asthma attacks are down.

Jacquelyn now eats more vegetables and whole grains and less red meat and sweets. She has also established a regular fitness schedule that begins at 5 A.M. four days a week. She puts on her workout gear, grabs a bottle of water, and heads for the gym that her husband has set up for her in their basement. This is HER time, exclusively for her to replace complacency with gusto.

The overall quality of her life has greatly improved. She looks great and feels great! She is a SUPER(IOR) WOMAN! Jacquelyn is PHIT4LIFE! Ladies, it doesn't matter if you are single or married with children, you can find the time to exercise if you're willing to make a commitment to change. Instead of just sitting and doing nothing while watching TV, get on your stationary bike or tread-mill, or try a set of sit-ups. Get up an hour earlier while everyone else is still asleep and get your exercise in, or exercise after putting the children to bed at night. Find time to replace fast-food meals with home-cooked meals by taking time out to cook a few days' worth of nutritious meals on the weekend. This is the time to give back to yourself so that you'll be able to be at your best for years to come!

11

THE FAT IS MELTING
AWAY BUT MY CLOTHES ARE
HANGING OFF

I'm proud to say that African-American women have a long tra-
dition of looking good no matter what their size. This is no time
to let your closet or your style hit the skids. Your body is changing.
Sometimes the change will be rapid and you'll experience a major
drop in weight. Other times it will seem like the weight and inches
are coming off at a snail's pace. You'll hit a plateau and think
you'll never lose another inch. If you're like me, your pocketbook
won't be able to keep up. Don't worry! One of the best-known
secrets in the retail fashion world today is the proliferation of
high-end resale shops. We are talking designer clothes at rock-bot-
tom prices.

Never believe that fat equals unattractive or thin equals beauty.
I've seen some of the most gorgeous women, who just happen to
be a plus size, catching the eye of more than one person as they
walk down the street. Some of these women did not necessarily
have beautiful faces, but they knew how to work their assets and

minimize their shortcomings. They had confidence and style to spare.

Studies have shown that over fifty-five percent of first impressions are based on appearance and actions. Within the first seven seconds of seeing someone, value judgments are made based solely on appearance, whether consciously or unconsciously. (*The Plus Size Guide to Looking Great.*) I decided while I was losing weight that I would slowly give myself a total makeover. I've seen so many women lose weight who never change their look, hair, or style of clothes, nor even add makeup. Not this sister! My goal was not only to lose weight and be healthy but to a transform myself into a stylish, sophisticated woman. I used to spend hours looking through fashion magazines just wishing I could look good enough to wear some of those sharp outfits. I was working hard on my inside as well as my outside so that I wasn't just going to look ordinary; I wanted to be stunning! This was my makeover wish list:

> Get rid of my perm damaged hair.
> Learn to stand and walk with correct posture.
> Stop walking slew-footed so the heels of my shoes
>   will last longer.
> Learn the art of applying makeup professionally.
> Wear clothes to compliment my complexion and
>   figure.

The first step I took was getting professional help with my hair. I needed a hairstyle that wouldn't require a hot curling iron after every workout. I was working out five times a week, sweating madly, and my hair was getting badly damaged and starting to look unprofessional. I started going to the African Braiding House and had elegant braids put into my hair. I also went to Cornrows & Co., a natural hair-care salon in Washington, D.C. to have a hair and scalp analysis done. I started training myself to walk straight without slumping.

Weight began to melt off my thighs, I walked straighter, my feet no longer looked like a penguin's, and the heels of my shoes stopped running down. I invested in three books by well-known makeup artists—Sam Fine, Reggie Wells, and Kevyn Aucoin. And finally, I purchased a book called *Plus Style—The Plus Size Guide to Looking Great.*

I learned how to choose the right accessories, how to mistake-proof my shopping for quality and fit, how to choose my best colors, and where to find plus-size stores, catalogs, and outlets. But best of all I identified my body type and what fashions complimented my figure best. So now when I go to the resale shops (of course I still go, why give up on a good thing?) I look for soft, flowing, or "drapeable" fabrics. I also look for slightly narrower skirts and tailored dresses to compliment my body type.

By the time I was able to fit into a size 16, I didn't have hundreds of dollars to spend on a whole new wardrobe. Instead, I went straight to my mother in Florida and then to my Auntie Vernell in Detroit. These two women have got to be the uncrowned queens of the designer resale shops. They had me looking like I should be on the cover of a magazine. I felt like a queen. Without a doubt, Mom and Auntie Vernell knew *the* best resale shops with *the* best clothes with *the* best prices. Before leaving Miami or Detroit, I had to buy another suitcase just to pack all my beautiful new clothes, not to mention the silk scarves, belts, and handbags that I picked up too. Now just in case you're sitting there thinking that a resale shop sounds tacky, well, girlfriend, think again. We buy pre-owned cars, we scour yard sales, and secondhand baby shops are just the ticket for new mothers. Why not take advantage of somebody else's good taste?

Look for these styles of clothes that will shrink with you as you lose weight:

Drawstring or elastic-waist pants • Knits

Surplice dresses • Jumper dresses • Boxy jackets

Raglan sleeves   •   Wrap skirts   •   Chemise dresses
Full set-in sleeves   •   Some coatdresses
Trapeze dresses

I also got great bargains when I shopped the malls at the end-of-season sales, sometimes getting anywhere from forty-to-seventy percent off the original price. The first year I lost all my weight, security had to escort me out of the mall because I had lost all track of time shopping in normal-sized clothing stores. When I wore a size 24, I hated going shopping, but today I can shop till I drop.

Another place to shop as you continue your meltdown is the local outlets. You can find some great bargains in the stores that specialize in plus sizes like Elisabeth, Jones New York Woman, and David Dart. I also found that shopping at outlets saved me quite a bit of money when it came to bras and underwear. When I started weight training, I lost inches so fast I couldn't stay in my bras and underwear for more than eight weeks.

Alterations are always part of weight loss, and if you can do them yourself you're that much ahead of the game. If sewing is not one of your gifts (and believe me, it's not mine), then find a good seamstress. Just remember, though, clothing can't be altered more than one size before your favorite outfit starts to lose its style and shape. Then it's time for you to pass it on.

And speaking of passing it on, this is a great opportunity for you to help others. One of my workshop members shared with us about places for plus-size women who literally cannot afford clothes but desperately need appropriate outfits for job interviews. These programs offer low-income women help in their efforts to achieve economic self-sufficiency by providing them with free interview attire and guidance in career development. The agencies offer workshops on résumé writing, interview skills, how to dress for an interview, and how to put together a working wardrobe. Women are referred from job-training programs, welfare-to-work programs, battered women's shelters, and halfway houses. They are given a complete outfit for their interview and, if they land the job, are invited back to get two or three more outfits. It's like a department store because you get to choose what you want, and there are "sales assistants" to help with accessories. Plus-size donations are *always* needed, so, ladies, as you melt down, you can help others by donating your now too-large wardrobe to the appropriate agency in your town, making a monetary donation, or volunteering to help.

HERE'S HOW YOU CAN HELP:

1. Clean your closet. Get rid of all those clothes and accessories you haven't worn during the past year and help change someone's life. Agencies can use:

   Interview-appropriate skirts, blouses, jackets, and
      dresses
   Shoes and handbags
   Scarves, belts, jewelry
   New, unopened pantyhose
   New, unopened cosmetics

2. Donate. Monetary gifts to most organizations are tax-deductible and many employers offer matching gift programs

   $25 will suit one person for a job interview
   $75 will suit three people
   $500 will suit a whole day of shoppers

3. Volunteer. Each organization has many volunteer opportunities. Contact one near you.

For a list of locations on the web, check www.dressforsuccess.org or ask at your local library. I know some great organizations in the northern Virginia/Washington, D.C., area that aren't listed on this site, so it pays to do a little investigating.

When the ladies from my workshop were having their after pictures taken for the book, a few of them were still wearing sizes that were too big for them. I told them it didn't make sense to lose weight if they were going to hide those new figures. If this is true for you too, then it's time to do some journal writing. Is there a reason you don't want to show off? Are you embarrassed by accomplishment? Think about it. Something is holding you back. Do you still see yourself overweight? I know it's hard to see that you are finally a smaller size, and sometimes it's hard to visualize that you may get even smaller. Ask someone who cares about your appearance if what you have on is flattering. As Alan Leo, our wonderful photographer, said, "You no longer have to buy clothes that compensate your figure. You're now buying clothes to accentuate your figure."

Okay ladies, I think I've got you covered from department stores to shopping for clothes free of charge. You're on your way to feeling good and lookin' good!

A journal entry describes my transformation while the journey continues.

August 25, 1995

> My wardrobe needs replacing. The size 20s and 18s are falling off me! Went shopping at the secondhand store. I'm wearing a size 16 at 190 pounds. I can't believe I'm wearing a size 16. But I read somewhere that when you lose the fat and build muscle through strength training, that muscle takes up less room than fat, therefore one can fit into a smaller size. My goodness, what size will I fit in when I reach my goal weight of 135 pounds?

November 23, 1995

It's going to be tough having Kelley here for the holidays. I know she will buy her favorite junk foods and bring it home. I have to make myself stay out of it. Kelley will be happy and shocked to see how much weight I've lost. We look so much alike now that the weight is coming off. Soon we will be able to share the same clothes like I've always dreamed.

November 24, 1995

Kelley is in town for the holidays and I love having her here! When she got off the plane and saw how much weight I had lost, she gasped. Then we screamed like two teenaged girls because I was starting to look so much like her. Kelley is thirty-five pounds lighter than I am right now and I always wished I could look like her. She has always been my mirror of what I could look like if I started loving myself. We went shopping at Nordstrom's for Dad's birthday present. He wanted a pair of shoes, so we browsed the shoe department. There was this tall beautiful dark-chocolate salesman asking if he could assist us. I assumed he was checking Kelley out, so I didn't pay him much attention. But when we were paying the bill and giving him the address of where to send the shoes, he started asking me questions. He asked if we were twins and if so, who was the oldest. I nearly fell out because people usually assume I'm the oldest (I am, by nine years). When we left the store Kelley told me how attracted he was to me. I haven't dated in so long or been around any testosterone that turned me on that I was clueless!! Hello!?

December 11, 1995

Today was so cold I didn't think I would ever get warmed up again. But the gentleman from Nordstrom warmed my heart by taking me to his favorite Chinese restaurant. I love the way he opens the car door for me when I'm getting in and out of the car. I love the way he takes my hand and guides me away from walking closest to the street. I love the way he helps me with my coat, taking it off and putting it on. But what I love best about him are the heart-warming messages he leaves on my answering machine, telling me what a wonderful evening he's had with me and how he can't wait to see me again. I don't erase the messages after listening to them because I love hearing them. Sometimes when I come home and I've had a trying day I'll listen to his messages and all is right with the world again. I know now that I can never accept anything less than a man like this, ever in my life again. He complements my life and doesn't complicate it like the other men I used to allow in my life.

December 15, 1995

Was not hungry for most of the day. Is it because I'm smitten by the man who sold me my father's shoes? I've never felt like this before! I exercised on the stepper for forty-five minutes. He's going to a Christmas party with me!

December 18, 1995

I'm so smitten by him, I'm forgetting to eat. I haven't behaved like this since I was a teenager. Today he told me he was moving back to the West Coast because he had a better chance of a promotion there. Even though I'm sad he's leaving, I'm glad I had the chance to meet a true gentleman. I believe God placed him in my life to set the standards of the type of men I should allow in my life.

December 26, 1996

Flew home to Miami for the holidays, and I'm 117 pounds lighter. The family is shocked and cannot believe how much weight I've lost. They haven't seen me at this weight since I was a teenager. The weather is beautiful and I went jogging around the neighborhood early this morning. I can't believe I'm jogging and I almost stopped to cry tears of joy, but managed to keep going. We went to see the movie *Waiting to Exhale* and it made me think of my former husband. The only way I was able to let go of the hate I had for him was to imagine him hanging from a tree by his balls. I have set fire underneath him like a campfire and have invited all my girlfriends that he hates over for this glorious occasion. We're sitting in a circle around him, singing songs from *Waiting to Exhale*. While we sing in unison, swaying back and forth to the rhythm, we're passing around a huge box of chocolates. Between each verse I'm yelling out to everyone which chocolates have caramel, cherry, and crème fillings while still keeping rhythm, like black men working on the railroad with their sledgehammers. I realized I was using food to release my pain like a small child, forever lying about stupid things. He used sex to release his pain and was forever trying to prove his manhood.

January 30, 1996

Even though things didn't work out between me and the man who sold me my father's shoes, I'm still thankful that I got to know him. I now know that it's possible for me to love again. Lord, the way he made me feel when we went to din-

ner. I adored the way he would reach out to hold my hand—
bring on the fans!

February 5, 1996

Today when I walked and passed a mirror, I had to take a
double take. I couldn't believe this was my reflection! I had
become another person mentally, physically, and spiritually. When I got home from work today, I took out all my
old before pictures along with my new after pictures. I
made an album with captions underneath each picture,
remembering the event when the picture was taken. I
looked at my wedding pictures. I was in a cream-colored
pleated skirt that was so tight I couldn't wait to get out of it
after saying "I do." I looked at the picture of me at 245
pounds, then me at 292 pounds. My whole body language
was different in those pictures compared to my after pictures. It's funny back then men didn't look my way. I don't
think it had to do with my weight totally because I've seen
some overweight sisters get lots of attention from the men.
It was the way I carried myself. I had no confidence in my
inner or outer beauty.

"Once you begin to view yourself positively, you can accept
and believe that passing stranger who gives you a sincere
compliment about your beauty. The inner beauty of your
soul will shine through so others may see. When I talk about
inner beauty it is the difference between a woman who walks
into a room full of people and is noticed for her fantastic
hairstyle or the woman who walks in and is remembered
because of her radiance and assured presence, where everything about her is beautiful. We have all seen this type of
beautiful woman and remember the little things as well as
the entire spirit. The love she exudes from within touches

many people who are searching for inner peace and beauty."
Let's Talk Hair, by Pamela Ferrell (Cornrows & Co. Publications/Washington, D.C.).

March 12, 1996

All day today I had to stop and pull my pantyhose up because they kept sagging at the ankles. I was also walking out of my shoes all day. When I talked to Mom this evening she said, "Girl, your pantyhose are probably too big as well as your shoes because you don't wear plus/queen size anymore!" It never occurred to me, but she was right! I went to Towson Town Center and brought a normal-sized pair of pantyhose and also had my feet measured. I was now wearing a size 8½ shoe instead of a size 10. The saleswoman looked at me as if I was crazy for wearing shoes that were too big.

April 16, 1996

It's Tuesday evening and I'm dangerous! I'm on my way to an evening at the Aquarium that my company is sponsoring. My gray wool suit (secondhand store find) fits just right and is perfect for this cool spring evening. My makeup is fresh and light and my glorious braids cascade down to my shoulders. I'm looking fierce! When I arrived, the parking lot attendant and waiters confirm my beauty by falling all over themselves to accommodate me. I feel like a QUEEN! The representatives from D.C., Virginia, and Delaware don't recognize me. When I walk up to them and say hello, they looked puzzled until I reintroduce myself. Everyone's mouth dropped open when they realized it's me! One of the girls I had a falling-out with sees me and nearly faints. She is pissed and shocked. I can tell from the look on her face and from her body language. Don't hate me because I'm beautiful!

The next two success stories in this chapter are from my sister and my aunt. I included them because it just proves that lifestyle changes can be a family affair and that it's never too late to get healthy.

Kelley Phillips

Age: 31—single
Children: none
Starting weight: 160 lbs.
Height: 5'6"
Weight lost: 30 lbs.
Inches lost: 19

My sister and best friend Kelley is just coming to terms with being slim. She discovered after attending one of my workshops that she had been afraid to be a perfect size 6 because of wanting to be accepted by female friends. I was shocked to learn that she had been sabotaging herself for years, keeping an extra ten, then twenty, then thirty pounds on her body to feel accepted by women in general. However, her first memory of overeating is not because of wanting to be accepted, but fear of missing out on her favorite foods.

Our oldest brother Roy, Junior, would often get up in the middle of the night and eat snacks and leftovers from the day's dinner. Kelley would be very disappointed the next day when she discovered that the food that she was looking forward to eating was gone. So she decided to eat as much as she could while it was there, thinking that she would probably never see it again. Kelley went on her first diet to lose five pounds when our mother said she was getting a little too thick. Mom told her to watch her intake of Funyuns (crispy onion-flavored chips) and candy that she bought after school. Kelley did lose weight, but from that point on would periodically gain and lose five pounds until junior high school. She was in junior high when she joined Weight Watchers with Mom to lose ten pounds. The women in the class were appalled that someone her age was joining Weight Watchers, but Kelley told them that she was there because she didn't want it to become a bigger problem. She lost weight and kept it off through high school. In high school Kelley was not comfortable with the fact that some of her female classmates seemed catty toward her at times—especially if she was wearing something to accent her figure and the guys noticed. That bothered her, but she understood enough to put two and two together.

In college Kelley gained fifteen pounds in her first year and noticed that no one acted catty toward her at all. As soon as she lost weight she noticed the girls were not as friendly, and one of them embarrassed her in front of the class. Kelley was passing out music to the choir and one of the jealous girls took Kelley by her arm and said, "Kelley, you're not planning on losing any more weight, are you? I mean you look fine, but PLEASE don't lose any more." Kelley instantly became self-conscious and noticed everyone looking at her. She knew that when men were looking at her, giving her admiring looks and compliments, it irritated some of the other girls in the choir. Kelley didn't feel comfortable with the attention she was getting from the men and certainly didn't like alienating the insecure girls in the choir. She wanted everyone to like her, not just her friends. It was at that point that she consciously decided to let herself go a little. And for the rest of her college career she repeatedly gained and lost ten pounds. It was a vicious cycle.

After finishing college, Kelley became really depressed because she didn't feel like she had anything to offer. She allowed her self-esteem to be stripped by some very negative people and professors who told her she wasn't talented. She believed them. Kelley moved to North Carolina with her fiancé and when she couldn't find a teaching job because she didn't apply early enough, she gained twenty pounds. She moved back home and told her fiancé she wanted to wait a year before they married because she wanted to experience life on her own first.

Kelley lost twenty pounds and was accepted to the number-one music school in the country for graduate studies. She was extremely lonely and depressed because five months earlier her fiancé had told her he didn't love her anymore. Our brother had died of AIDS two years before and she still hadn't dealt with it. Kelley's weight fluctuated between 135 and 155 pounds throughout graduate school. In fact, after her first year, she pretty much stayed around one hundred and fifty pounds.

Finally, Kelley got sick and tired of being sick and tired and decided to get on with her life. She met someone new in her last year of school. She finally felt intelligent and knew she had something to offer the music world. Unfortunately, her extra pounds had become part of her lifestyle and she stopped caring about her weight. Everyone at school knew her at that weight and had nothing to compare it to. Kelley had a very stressful job teaching inner-city kids and really began to eat. She was now up to 160 pounds—the highest weight she had ever been. She also suffered with uterine fibroids and was very anemic, leaving her in pain—too dizzy and tired to exercise.

She saw and knew how I was losing weight and was terrified that when she came home for Christmas, she would be bigger than me. Well, her worst nightmare came true. She thought the whole family would say something about her weight gain and was very ashamed. No one said anything and she asked me what I had done to lose weight. Kelley followed my advice—all except for keeping a diary to find out why she was overeating—and lost thirty pounds, but she hadn't dealt with the reasons why she was overeating, why she was so uncomfortable being a healthy size 6.

After she lost thirty pounds, Kelley was so self-conscious she couldn't even walk straight without bumping into things. She always had at least one bruise on her. Kelley decided to attend my workshops not as my sister, but as a client. She didn't think that she was in the same boat as the other women in class because she wasn't obese. Her attendance dropped and she gained all of her weight back within a matter of four months.

Kelly finally said enough is enough and became a regular member of my workshops. She followed my suggestion and started keeping a journal. Finally she lost thirty pounds for good. One day she noticed how flat her stomach was looking and panicked. Silly Kelley was terrified of having a flat stomach. I told her to write about it in her journal and she shared it with the class and worked through it.

Now, a year later, Kelley is still in a size 6 and finally knows it's an okay place to be. Little does Kelley know she has always been my mirror, helping me to visualize what I could look like if I learned to trust and love myself. Thank you, sister!

Vernell Ingram

Age: 56—divorced
Mother of three sons (30, 33, 37 years), one daughter (31 years)
Grandmother of four
Starting weight: 258 lbs.
Height: 5'4"
Weight lost to date: 40 lbs.
Inches lost: 28

My Aunt Vernell was always very thin as a child, and during her early and middle teens. Her weight problem started after her mother died—she was nineteen years old and had a two-year-old son. She was feeling totally abandoned. Food soothed her and made her feel better.

Four years later, Aunt Vernell married. There were a lot of

problems in the marriage, and they separated six years and three children later. Again she felt abandoned. This time she was alone with four children at the age of twenty-nine. Her weight slowly escalated out of control and she felt powerless to stop it.

I've seen Aunt Vernell lose hundreds of pounds through the years, attending weight-loss classes, taking shots and pills, but regaining it all back and more. The more she gained, the more she ate and the worse she felt—a vicious cycle.

In 1983, Aunt Vernell developed high blood pressure; in 1991, asthma; in 1994, diabetes; and in 1995, breast cancer. She was only fifty-one years old and needed comfort—something to rid her of the pain of all these illnesses. She felt her whole world seemed to revolve around her next food fix. She would become euphoric for the moment, but like the typical food addict, she would soon feel disgusted and hate herself. Then food would be the only thing to give her peace—and the cycle continued off and on until June of 1999.

In June, Aunt Vernell went to see her sister, who is also diabetic. Her sister could barely walk, and it took approximately three to five minutes for her to get from her bed to the door. Aunt Vernell knew she didn't want to be this way. She knew she didn't want to become like her. The next day her sister could not walk, could not even get out of bed. Aunt Vernell had to attend to her as if she were a baby, changing her, bathing her, and giving her medicine— so many pills! When Aunt Vernell left, she was devastated and sad that they were putting her sister in a home where someone could take care of her twenty-four hours a day.

When Aunt Vernell returned home, she called me and vowed to start exercising and eating better. I was shocked because she started eating better right away.

Thank God she finally did incorporate exercise—walking! Aunt Vernell went back to the doctor a month later and her blood sugar was down for the first time since she was diagnosed with diabetes.

Her sugar level had run between 400 and 500 and was now down to 124, and this was before she started seriously exercising!

She now consistently walks two miles a day, six days a week. To date she has lost forty pounds and has vowed to keep eating healthy and exercising—even when she doesn't feel like moving. Her legs have ached for years and the doctor told her to walk and they would feel better. She didn't believe him but has come to know that it is, indeed, true. The ache has dissipated a lot and she's feeling better and stronger each day. When I speak to my Aunt Vernell on the phone she says she will not give up, and cannot give up until she reaches the other side of the bulge. She knows her freedom and health depend on it. Keep going, Aunt Vernell, I know you can do it!

This just proves that no matter how old you are, no matter what illness you suffer from, and no matter how stressful your job may be, you can turn your life around and begin to change. It's never too late to start exercising and eating right and you can possibly even prolong your life if you choose to start today. Let your meltdown begin today and watch your clothes start hanging. But don't forget to donate those clothes.

12

CONGRATULATIONS! YOU JUST BETTER GO, GIRL!

*L*ook at you now. You are fine, fit, and fabulous, and need a bodyguard to keep the men away. This is the time to understand and incorporate techniques for maintaining your weight loss and mental peace. Believe me, you have not only lost fat and inches but also years of emotional baggage, tons of negativity, and a lifetime of putting yourself at the end of the line.

I had to learn to feel comfortable in my new body, and so will you. When I was a little girl, one of my mother's friends lost over sixty pounds. She then intentionally gained every pound back because she said she was uncomfortable in her new body, and others were, too. Mom and I thought she looked terrific when she was thin, and I could never understand why someone who looked so good would destroy all that hard work. Just think of the effort and commitment it took to lose those sixty pounds. Mom tried to explain the fear of success, but back then I just didn't get it.

But today it's all Crystal-clear. After I reached a healthy weight, I felt very uncomfortable. I was clumsy, always tripping over myself, with men staring and women glaring. I struggled a little, afraid of having all the attention I wasn't used to. Part of me wanted to disappear again. Never in my wildest dreams did I imagine I'd be in this predicament. I used to have fantasies about how wonderful I'd feel and look after losing weight. I envisioned myself walking down the street looking beautiful and feeling on top of the world. My inner and outer glow would be so bright, people would stop in their tracks and wonder, "Who's that girl?" Cars would crash into one another and into fire hydrants because the drivers just couldn't take their eyes off the new ME! Hey, this was my *fantasy*, okay?

Anyway, something like that did happen one spring day. I was going into the post office in downtown Baltimore wearing one of my beautiful secondhand outfits. As I made my way to the front door of the building, a man who was coming out stopped and walked back, trying to open the front door for me. I was only carrying a small purse, so I was confused and he looked a little embarrassed as I entered the electronic doors instead that were automatically opening. He looked like he was headed for work because he was dressed in an expensive business suit and getting into a very expensive car. No, this was no wino with nothing else to do.

Next, another man who was standing in front of me in line was summoned by the next free postal clerk to her end of the counter to be served. When he saw me behind him, he smiled and motioned for me to take his turn. I thought maybe he wanted to do business with a particular postal clerk until I saw him step up and simply buy stamps with no conversation. When he passed me he nodded his head, smiled, and gave me a look of approval and respect.

Now, ya'll, I'm a conservative dresser when I go to work. I'm not one of those people who lose their mind after losing weight and start wearing crazy, skintight, short, revealing outfits. I was wearing a conservative royal-blue silk suit. The skirt hit just above the knee and I was wearing sensible black leather two-inch heels. I panicked at all the attention and immediately headed for the bathroom, thinking either my boobs were hanging out or my skirt was tucked up into my panty hose in the back. I just wasn't used to having men give me so much attention. When I finally looked in the mirror, nothing was out of place—except my brain. I was not used to seeing myself at this weight and couldn't believe I was wearing a size 6 suit. I had *never* before worn a size 6 as an adult. I had to retrain my brain to accept me at a normal weight.

Did I truly want life without pain? How would I remain balanced and not become too involved in the new me? Would I be one of the ninety-seven percent who gain their weight back after two years? Could I be truly happy and go for all I wanted after years of rejection and second-guessing myself? When all the people who cheered me on had gone on with their lives, would they expect more and different things from me? Would I always feel slightly attacked when someone complimented my body? Would I always feel slightly scared by flattery? What new problems would I encounter at this new weight? I knew what to expect when I was fat, but what about now? What would I do now?

The answer is simple. Constantly surround yourself with winners, people who are confident and supportive and want the best for you and from you. These are the people who will teach you how to accept success instead of pulling you down like a crab in a boiling pot of hot water. In Overeaters Anonymous, some meetings are designed for "maintainers." That is the sole focus and agenda of these meetings, to help you endure the "stress of success" and "problems of abundance." I'll never forget one of my first OA meetings. I said I was afraid to become a normal size again. Someone told me to become a normal size first, then talk about taking the next step. He was right. I had to stop examining the struggle until I was there in the moment of that struggle. I felt like a newborn learning how to walk again, but this time I was determined to tolerate success and avoid returning to the familiarity of failure. In a way, staying in your addiction is the perfect way to avoid growing up, to stay at home forever. But now that I have completed building my beautiful new brick house, I don't want to go back to the old place. I've lived in fear and contemplated suicide. NOW IT'S TIME TO FLY!

Crystal's 10 Steps for Maintenance

1. If you are starting to gain weight or are getting out of the healthy eating pattern that has helped you to lose and maintain your weight for a while, don't ignore this problem. Identify the problem by talking it out and writing it out as soon as possible. Know when you're lapsing or relapsing.

2. You've fought hard to save your life, now get a life and start doing fun things. Get involved in charitable causes, serve as a mentor to a young girl or boy in need, and volunteer for something at church or work. Give back to the world and the world will support you.

3. Identify a source of constant stress and rid yourself of it or minimize it quickly. If there is more than one source of stress, work it out one at a time.

4. Never resort to dieting. You're only setting yourself up for deprivation, sabotage, and an eventual weight gain.

5. Accept who you are, body type and all. Don't stress or mess with tripping over what a magazine or TV commercial or newspaper says you should look like. You've come too far to fall into that game again.

6. Open yourself to love. Don't hold the brothers at bay just because you've been hurt. Remember that you have arrived as a queen, and now you will attract a king. Love your sisters, too: as women you share a bond that can never be broken.

7. Stay honest and move out of the blindness of denial.

8. If your eating and your exercise plans no longer fit your lifestyle, revise them to suit you
9. Never be afraid to seek professional help or go back to what gives you peace, strength, courage, and faith.
10. Never let the scale alone be your judge. The fit of your clothes and your behavior toward exercise and food should always be your guide.

Check out this journal entry.

June 11, 1996

Today I've dressed slowly and carefully and have applied my makeup just so. I'm meeting my former husband and his fiancée at the mortgage company today so he can refinance our home in his name. When they walked in he looked around wondering where I was and asked the loan officer if I was running late. I can't believe he doesn't recognize me sitting by the loan officer. (The loan officer has no idea that I lost all this weight and is looking at my former husband like he's crazy.) When I tell him I'm here, his mouth dropped. I wish I had a camera because this was truly a Kodak moment. He hadn't seen me since I left him (September 23, 1993, 8:39 A.M.). His fiancée said, "I thought you told me she was fat!" There was silence and she turned very stern and started reading Scriptures from the Bible silently after they sat down.

13

PASSING IT ON

I told you at the beginning that I was here to stay and now I'll help you start your support group to break the cycle of obesity and expand the Sister Circle. The Through Thick & Thin™ workshop is two eight-week programs designed to help you examine your eating behaviors. The goal is to help you resolve why you eat when you are not physically hungry and build a plan of action to overcome behaviors that are harmful to you mentally as well as physically. Through Thick & Thin™ is not a diet program. It is a program for lifestyle change and is designed to help you lose weight by approaching compulsive eating as a symptom of a bigger problem.

It's simple to start your own Through Thick & Thin™ workshop support group. If you belong to a church, sorority, book club, or any other organization, you've got a great place to begin. The workplace and your neighborhood associations are other ideal places to find women who are interested in change. You aren't looking for a whole gang of people, you just need to find one or two others who are committed to being healthy.

The bad news is I can't meet with every one of you personally. The good news is I can outline for you everything we do here in my hometown workshops. You can also E-mail me or visit my Web site at www.crystalphillips.com.

First, decide when and where you are going to meet. Maybe it will be in someone's home or at church or maybe even the local community center. Set a time and stick to it. This is part of your lifestyle change.

Second, start by discussing the entire program. No one should be surprised or uncomfortable about what is expected.

Third, take time to do the following. Be honest, not judgmental.

- Use a camera for before and after pictures
- Take your measurements once a month
- Weigh in the first week and use the same scale to weigh at the end of week four and week eight
- Use printed forms to record everyone's weight and measurements

And now, lets get started.

Week 1 Overview

AFTER INTRODUCTIONS discuss your individual and group goals. Talk about lifestyle changes rather than pounds lost. Take before pictures; chart everyone's measurements, and weigh in. Do both once a month. Discuss why you would like to lose weight in terms of your health. Read over the topics you will be discussing over the next eight weeks.

Week 2 Overview

FIND THE ROOT OF YOUR PROBLEM AND ACCEPT WHO YOU ARE TODAY Discuss your first memory of when and why you began using food to give you comfort and companionship. Look at both sides of your family. Who else is overweight in your family? This is the time to sit down with your family and tell them that you will need their support in order to make your lifestyle change successful. What do you need from your family in order to make your lifestyle transition easier?

Start to think positively about yourself by looking in the mirror and pointing out what you like about yourself and your body. Affirmations are healing and allow you to accept yourself—flaws and all. Create a positive affirmation about yourself. Repeat your affirmation daily while looking in the mirror. Do it *before* you leave your house in the morning. This will help you to keep a positive internal dialogue and eliminate negative self-talk. Remember to face your feelings instead of feeding your emotions.

List five ways to deal with your feelings instead of *eating* over your feelings:

1.
2.
3.
4.
5.

Week 3 Overview

BUILD A STRONG FOUNDATION FOR YOUR MOTIVATION Discuss what will motivate you for the long haul. Unlike a diet, this is a lifestyle change. You must stay committed for the rest of your life if you want the weight to stay off permanently. Don't let that scare you before you even get started. You will feel so good—mentally and physically—that you won't even think about not being committed. How have you tried to lose weight before? Why didn't it work for you? Eating *sensibly* and exercising *regularly* is the key to permanent weight loss. Discuss the pros and cons of exercise as it relates to you. Now discuss solutions to the cons of exercising on a regular basis.

- What are you willing to do to be healthy?
- Will you let your hair come between you and your health? How can you overcome the challenge of keeping up with your hair after you work out three to six times a week?
- How will you incorporate exercise into your schedule? If you are a single parent, how will you overcome the sitter problem when you are attending to your health?

This may also be a good time to pick an exercise buddy. Based on your weight and past activity levels, what exercise will be best suited for you? If you suffer from back and/or knee problems, discuss what exercises you can still do safely. Does anyone in the group know about aqua aerobics?

For the next class, prepare to bring a *tasty* nutritious dish. Don't forget to type up the recipe with calories and fat-gram counts—it's good to know nutritional values. And make a copy for everyone in class.

Week 4 Overview

BUILDING BLOCKS—WHAT TO EAT AND THE IMPORTANCE OF DRINKING WATER Before starting, take measurements and weigh in. Chart everyone's progress. This is a great time to share your low-fat dishes. Since this is not a diet program, talk about what foods satisfy you mentally and physically. Look at the food pyramid and discuss how you will balance your meals so they are more nutritious for you and your family. Discuss how you will handle eating at work, traveling on business or on vacation, or eating at a restaurant. Why is it so important to drink at least eight glasses of water a day?

Week 5

GETTING HONEST TO BE FREE What strategies will you use to help you stay honest about what you eat and why you eat when you're not hungry? What time do you eat your regular meals? Do you even eat regular meals, or do you snack all day?

Discuss five strategies you will use to avoid eating when you're not hungry.

1.
2.
3.
4.
5.

Week 6

DAMN IT! I WANTED IT, SO I ATE IT! Discuss how to retrain that spoiled child within and how to recognize the silent sounds and screams of sabotage. What strategies will you incorporate to deal with high-risk food situations like holiday parties, Halloween, birthdays, weddings, and even funerals?

Name five ways to deal with overeating on those special occasions

1.
2.
3.

4.
5.

Week 7

WEIGHT STRENGTH TRAINING Bring in a certified personal trainer to discuss the benefits of strength training with light weights. (They are not that hard to find and, yes, they would love to talk with you.) Talk about how your clothes are starting to fit since you've started your lifestyle change. What are you doing to keep your wardrobe shrinking with you? Are you looking good?

Week 8 Congratulations

YOU'VE COMPLETED EIGHT WEEKS! Take measurements and weigh each member.

If you have reached your weight-loss goal, congratulations! This is the time to understand and incorporate techniques for maintaining your weight loss and mental peace. This is also a great time to talk about the differences between lapses and relapses. Members who wish to continue for another eight weeks can also discuss the above and the new topics that will follow in the next eight weeks.

What is a lapse?

What is a relapse?

Week 9

PHYSICAL HUNGER VERSUS EMOTIONAL HUNGER How do you determine if you are physically hungry or emotionally hungry? What techniques have you developed to help you to avoid eating when you're just emotionally hungry? Discuss "good foods" and "bad foods" and how you plan to incorporate foods that you consider bad foods back into your life so you will not feel deprived.

Week 10

PORTION CONTROL Do you know what a portion or one serving size looks like? Have on hand a fat-gram/calorie book and look at what the serving sizes are for the following:

- Meat
- Vegetables
- Fruits
- Milk
- Starch/Breads
- Desserts/Sweets

Discuss the psychology of leaving food on your plate. Learn to use your hand for portion control. The *palm* of your hand (not the whole thing) is approximately the size of a meat serving. Your thumbnail is about a teaspoon.

Week 11

RECOVERY Discuss how you would help others to recover from an overeating episode. Devise a plan of how to overcome an overeating episode in the future. Discuss what triggered the overeating episode. Use your imagination. Be prepared.

Week 12

SELF-NURTURING Take measurements and weigh in. Chart everyone's progress. Discuss how to become gentler with your body and your emotions. How do you relax after an awful, awful day? Do you take a bubble bath, exercise, or go to a day spa? Or do you eat? Learn to take care of yourself without feeding your feelings with food. Name five ways to de-stress and nurture yourself:

1.

2.

3.

4.

5.

Week 13

WHAT IS YOUR EATING BEHAVIOR? Discuss these four eating behaviors:

- Starver—Restricts calories to the extreme until weight loss occurs rapidly.
- Binger—Eats large quantities of food within a short period of time.
- Purger—Rids the body of unwanted food and calories after eating.
- Grazer—Eats unhealthy foods from morning to evening without having a set meal time.

Which one describes you and what have you done to seek help?

Week 14

KEEP EXERCISING Have you continued to incorporate exercise into your week? If you are on any medication, have you been able to reduce the amount of medication you're taking because you have continued eating and exercising regularly? How are people starting to respond to the new you? Have you changed or added to your exercise routine? Are you loving it yet?

Week 15

BODY IMAGE Discuss how you're feeling about your body after fifteen weeks. What changes do you see? Discuss with your doctor what a healthy goal weight will be for you. Visualize what you want for yourself as you build on your new lifestyle. Will you go out more? Do you want to learn how to swim? Is it time to look for a new job? What about dating? Does it feel good to be getting attention?

Name five things you've always wanted to do but never did because you felt your weight was in the way.

1.
2.
3.
4.
5.

Week 16

CHANGING TO A BETTER YOU! CONGRATULATIONS! Take an after picture, your measurements, and your weight. Change is a never-ending journey. How will you stay committed to your new lifestyle? Discuss how the group will continue to meet for those who want to lose more weight and for those who would like to maintain their healthy weight and lifestyle. Start another group and pass it on.

July 4, 1996

> I jumped out of bed this morning so Heru and I can get an early-morning walk before the humidity becomes overbearing. I also weight-trained at home for thirty minutes. I'm feeling good and go to a cookout at a neighbor's house. My

neighbor makes ribs almost as good as my brother Roy's (nobody can touch his). I used to eat a slab by myself and my neighbor came pretty close. His wife used to look at us both horrified. This year I ate two bones with a plateful of his wife's wonderful fresh cucumber salad, my mom's low-fat buttermilk cornbread, and a grilled potato. He was disappointed that I didn't eat more and asked how they tasted. I told him the ribs were wonderful as usual, but I couldn't eat a whole slab even if I wanted to. I also reminded him of my new healthy lifestyle. By the time dessert was served I was satisfied and passed!

AND FINALLY—
WRITE ME! SEND ME PICTURES!
TELL ME ABOUT YOUR SUCCESS!
I WANT TO HEAR FROM YOU!

So many have written me already to share with me their success stories. They could be included in my next book and you can be too.

Write: Crystal Phillips
        P.O. Box 765
        Ellicott City, MD 21041-0765
E-mail: Crystalight59735@AOL.com

EPILOGUE

SUMMER 1999 When my parents adopted my four younger brothers and sisters in 1992, I knew they were going to have their hands full. After meeting them I knew the trouble would be even worse than I imagined. As soon as I heard my father's voice on my answering service, I knew there had been another death in the family. I could barely understand him because his voice was so heavy and filled with grief. I was sad and, at the same time, relieved when my father finally managed to say that my little sister Angela had died earlier in the morning. I was stunned: it had happened so quickly. I sat in shock for twenty minutes, saying over and over, "She was only sixteen years old." Angela had been sent home to die after her cardiologist told my parents there was nothing else he could do for her in the hospital. She suffered from many things, but bingeing and purging ended her life. Numerous complications had developed as a result of Angela's eating disorder— an enlarged heart, damage to her reproductive system and intestinal tract, cardiac arrhythmias, electrolyte imbalance, constipation, fatigue, muscle weakness, and depression. And she suffered with bipolar disorder.

Mom said that morning Angela was the first one up to eat breakfast. She went to the bathroom afterward, started purging, and then went back to bed. My mother and little brother could hear her while they prepared their own breakfast. Angela was dead when the hospice nurse arrived.

Before coming to my parents, Angela had known only pain and destruction. She had been sexually, physically, and mentally abused—all before her second birthday. Mom and Dad sought endless treatment for her, but she fought hard against accepting love or help from anyone.

The last time I saw Angela she was so thin, she could barely take five steps without getting tired. After losing my 157 pounds and being so proud, I admit I flirted with the idea of purging to get rid of the few pounds I had gained while writing the first chapter of this book. But I was too afraid I would become addicted. I knew how out of control I could be about my weight. Angela's death was a wake-up call.

I felt guilty for being so hard on Angela about everything. She was amazingly talented and had a gift for drawing beautiful things. She was bright and intelligent and excelled in school when she wasn't acting out. She could have soared through high school and college if she wanted. All those things that did not come easily for me I wanted for her. And I wanted her to want them, too.

When Angela began to threaten suicide, my parents sought assistance for her, and finally, after much discussion, placed her in a residential treatment center where her educational and psychological needs could be met. The medication diagnosed for her bipolar disorder resulted in a sixty-five pound weight gain. Then her heart condition was diagnosed and she lost weight. I know her self-esteem was almost nonexistent and I often wondered if my own weight loss had triggered something in her. Did she see gaining and losing weight as a way to gain attention? Was it her way of having some control over her life? Did she think it would protect her from being hurt again?

Just as we were leaving for the funeral, I learned that Angela would be buried next to Kevin. I had chosen not to be physically present at Kevin's funeral. I had spent too much time walking in the shadows with him and needed to say good-bye by myself and in my own way. What would I do now? What could I do now? I sang at Angela's funeral with a clear head and heart. She had been loved and would be loved still. She would be with my beloved Kevin and my Aunt Delores. She would have the peace she so desperately wanted. I'm thankful for having had Kevin and Angela in my life and, in many ways, they have saved my life.

Although I have finally reached the other side of the bulge, I still struggle. I still want to eat when I'm stressed, angry, bored, or deliriously happy. I still use prayer and journal writing. I talk with my family and with the dynamic women who come to my workshops and share in the Sister Circle. I exercise. I work at staying grounded and thankful.

Writing this book was bittersweet for me. It took everything I had to write the first two chapters. It was painful and enormously depressing to remember the passing of my brother, of his companion, and my Aunt Delores. I wanted to eat, but how could I? I needed to write. I needed to share my story. The rest of the book was God's grace. It energized me, comforted me, and inspired me. I hope it has done the same for you.

Please share this book with anyone you know who is struggling with their weight and support them in their efforts. Save a life and pass it on to the next generation.

Last but not least, here's a success story in progress from a woman who is very near and dear to my heart. She is my mentor and best friend: my mother.

Vira Phillips

Age: 62—Married
Mother of two sons (42 years, and one deceased at
33 years) two daughters (31 and 40 years).
Adopted four children from the same family: two
sons (13 and 14 years), two daughters (15 and one
deceased at 16 years).
Grandmother of one
Starting weight: 252 lbs.
Height: 5'5"
Weight lost to date: 17 lbs.
Inches lost: 12

Mom started gaining weight after her first pregnancy in 1958. She was a newlywed and away from her family for the first time in her life. Mom and her sisters were very close and she missed them tremendously. Dad was a graduate student and worked part-time. When he was home, he had to study and Mom was very lonely and used food to keep her company. After the birth of Mom's first child, she lost thirty pounds of the fifty she had gained. Then she became pregnant for the second and third time and kind of gave up on her weight.

She has lost many pounds though the years and gained them all back, and then more. Mom's weight has ranged from 150 lbs to 252 pounds in the forty-two years she's been married. While talking to me about her weight problem, Mom has come to know that she has a feeling of abandonment, but cannot remember when or why the feeling originated. She also remembers being frightened a lot as a child but can't remember why. She does know that food made her feel better—for the moment. She felt horrible about overeating and vowed not to let it happen again, but kept repeating the cycle over and over.

After the birth of Mom's fourth child (Kelley) in 1969, she

developed hypertension. Her doctor said that if she lost weight she probably would not have to take medication. But thirty years later she still must take medication.

Mom realizes that she has had many life changes within the past thirteen years. In 1986, Mom and Dad discovered Roy, Junior, was on crack and that Kevin was gay. The gay aspect did not bother Mom in the least, but she still remembers her response to Kevin when he told her. She immediately asked, "What about the AIDS virus?" The possibility of him contracting the virus hung over Mom and Dad like a dark cloud. Discovering that Roy, Junior, was taking crack was not a complete surprise. Still, it was a heartbreaking moment and Mom and Dad gave Roy, Junior, an ultimatum of going into treatment or leaving their home. Thank God he chose the former. Mom and Dad attended family counseling sessions with him and he made it through. To date, he has not looked back and is still clean.

Unfortunately, Kevin was not so lucky.

In 1989, Kelley went away to college. This was a huge adjustment because they were very close, but Mom had started to prepare herself for it the year before. Still, it was a difficult adjustment for her.

In 1992, my parents adopted four children—six, seven, eight, and nine years old. They were siblings and came to Mom and Dad with many problems. Approximately a month after they adopted them, Kevin died. In August of that year, Hurricane Andrew roared through the city. My parent's house was damaged extensively and they had to live in a trailer in back of the house for nine months before repairs were finished. In April 1993, Mom's youngest sister died, a month before they moved back into the house.

Near the end of 1997, the oldest adopted daughter contracted a severe heart condition. She was not a candidate for a heart transplant because of her mental condition. She died in the summer of 1999 at the age of 16.

Mom recognizes the stress she was under after they adopted the children and when her sister died. When Kevin and Aunt Delores died, she was not quite as stressed out because she knew their chances of survival were poor. Writing about all of the changes has made Mom realize how stressed she was and still is today. Changes are stressful, and eating is one way she deals with stress, loneliness, and the feelings of abandonment and fear in her life.

Mom knows she has to take one day at a time, sometimes one hour at a time. When Mom started, she lost thirty-seven pounds but has gained back twenty since the death of my adopted sister. Even though Mom does not know the origins of some of the issues that face her, she continues to work at becoming healthier. When I talk to her on the phone once a week, she tells me she is continuing to eat better and is exercising five to six days a week. She knows all her problems have not evaporated, but she's learning that food will not make them go away.

Mom has always been my role model and best friend, and I love her and Dad so much and feel blessed to have them both. They stood by my side as I talked to them about all the childhood fears and resentments I had. Thank God they always left a door open for me to come back. I will do all I can to extend their lives because I am grateful to them for giving me life.

Well, this is how I lost my excess baggage and how I helped others through my workshop. Now this is the time to make your lifestyle change and become healthier so that you can live a longer, more productive life. Much success and God bless!

RECIPES FOR THE SOUL

Mama's Buttermilk Cornbread

I went from a size 24 to a size 6 by changing the medicine cabinet in my mind.

INGREDIENTS

    1 cup of cornmeal mix
    1 cup nonfat buttermilk (pour for desired consistency)
    ½ teaspoon salt or sea salt
    1 egg

Preheat oven to 350–375°F. Mix together ingredients for one minute. Lightly grease 14x10 inch pan with butter or soy margarine. Let pan warm in oven until butter or soy margarine has melted. Pour mixture into pan. Bake at 350–375°F. until golden brown.

4 SERVINGS

    1 serving: 5 fat grams,
    140 calories

Sistah Woman's Naked Stir-Fried Greens

I call my little sister Kelley "Sistah Woman" because she can cook circles around me. One day I had a taste for some good ol' collard greens but without all the fat. Since it was hot outside that day, I didn't feel like eating any meat, so I told Sistah Woman to hold the meat. Sistah Woman marched right into the kitchen and created this wonderful, tasty dish that touched my soul. This is one dish that will make you go back for seconds like I did that day. This dish is low in fat but still tastes g-o-o-d!

INGREDIENTS

  1 large sweet onion, chopped
  3 fresh garlic cloves, grated
  1 lb. red chard, chopped
  1 lb. of cleaned chopped collard greens
  1 lb. of cleaned chopped kale greens
  2 teaspoons sea salt or regular table salt
  3½ teaspoons canola oil

Heat the oil in a large pot or wok set on medium-high heat. Add garlic and onions and cook until onions are translucent. Add kale and collard greens, along with 2 teaspoons salt. Stir until greens cook down, then let simmer for 5 minutes on medium high, stirring occasionally. Continue to simmer on low for 10 minutes and serve. Traditionally I know we must have meat in our greens and there's nothing wrong with that as long as you don't add fatback or ham hocks—too much fat! Remember, if you want to dress your "naked" greens, add a meat you like that is low in fat.

4 SERVINGS
  1 serving (1 cup): 12.25 fat grams, 154 calories

Kelley's Tantalizing Tuna

I've learned not to let others determine my weight. If they are insecure with my inner and outer beauty and glow, they now must adjust their eyes to my light.

— *Kelley, who lost thirty pounds.*

INGREDIENTS

2 2.5-oz. cans of all-natural albacore tuna packed in spring water, partially drained
6 regular or organic spring onions, chopped finely
3 regular or organic extra-large eggs
1 teaspoon salt or sea salt (if sodium-sensitive, skip this ingredient)
1 teaspoon white pepper
4 heaping teaspoons canola mayonnaise (use less according to personal preference)

Simmer eggs for 10 minutes or until hard-boiled.

Break up the chunks of tuna until all chunks disappear.

Add onions, and white pepper.

Chop boiled eggs finely and add to tuna.

Add canola-oil mayonnaise and mix all ingredients until well blended.

5 SERVINGS

1 serving (½ cup): 6 fat grams, 62 calories

Add some great-tasting whole-wheat crackers, bread, or pasta.

Fresh Turkey Necks and Cabbage

Surrendering to God, my higher power, and doing His work with sweat and tears, I'm now carrying a lighter load.

INGREDIENTS

2 large heads of fresh-washed and chopped cabbage
8 to 10 chopped fresh-washed turkey necks
3 large onions, chopped
2 bell peppers, chopped
3 or 4 bundles of celery, chopped
2 tablespoons seasoned salt
2 teaspoons white or black pepper
2 packets of Equal
½ gallon of water

Put turkey necks into a large pot. Season with salt and pepper and cover with 1⁄2 gallon of water (taste to see if the seasonings are to your liking). Cook until tender, about 21⁄2 hours.

Pour broth into a large pot with the toughest green layers (usually top layers) of the cabbage and cook for 15 minutes. Then add the rest of the cabbage, the white part of the cabbage, together with bell pepper, celery, and 2 packets of Equal. Simmer for about 25 minutes. When cabbage is ready, combine turkey necks and vegetables. For a fuller flavor, let dish sit overnight in refrigerator.

10 SERVINGS

1 serving (1 cup cabbage and 4 ounces turkey): 9 fat grams, 229 calories

This is a great dish if you're having a houseful of people. It's light on the pocketbook, too!

Mama's Sugar-Free Banana Pudding

An estimated 3 million African-Americans have diabetes, which adds up to one in every ten of us. We are fifty-five percent more likely than whites to have diabetes, and the disease is especially prevalent in older black women. According to many experts, half of all patients don't even know they have it.

Diabetes runs in my family. My father and Aunt Vernell have type-2 diabetes (diagnosed in their late forties or early fifties), which is the most common, especially among African-Americans. My father's diabetes is being controlled without insulin because he controls his weight with new eating habits and exercise. Since diabetes is such a problem for so many in my family, Mama came up with this delicious sugar-free banana pudding. At first I was real leery 'cause I love my sweets, and banana pudding has always been one of my favorites, especially Mama's. But when I took that first spoonful, it was all over with. It tasted like the real thing. So with Mama's permission, I would like for you to try her life-saving creation.

INGREDIENTS

    40 to 45 sugar-free vanilla wafers
    7 to 8 medium-ripe bananas, sliced
    12 packets of Equal
    ¼ cup all-purpose flour
    ½ teaspoon salt
    2 eggs, separated
    2 cups 1-percent milk
    ½ teaspoon vanilla extract
    Set aside 10 to 14 vanilla wafers and one banana for top layer.

Combine Equal, flour, and salt in large nonstick pot. Stir in egg yolks and milk; blend well. Cook, uncovered, stirring continuously, for 5 minutes, or until thickened. Remove from heat, stir in vanilla extract. Spread small amount on bottom of 1½ quart casserole dish; cover with layer of vanilla wafers. Top with layer of sliced bananas. Pour about one-third of custard over bananas. Continue to layer wafers, bananas, and custard to make 3 layers each, ending with custard. Garnish with reserved banana slices and sugar-free vanilla wafers. Let cool or chill before serving.

10 SERVINGS

serving (1 cup): 8 fat grams, 350 calories

Crystal's Apple-Banana Pancakes

I had to find a new way of viewing and accepting exercise as a part of my life. Now I view exercise as a gift I give to myself each morning.

INGREDIENTS

1½ cups Arrowhead Mills Multi-Grain Pancake and
Waffle Mix
1 cup 1-percent milk *or* vanilla-almond non-dairy
beverage or soy non-dairy beverage
½ teaspoon nutmeg
½ teaspoon cinnamon
1 medium mashed banana
¼ cup sugar-free or organic applesauce
1 teaspoon butter or soy margarine

Heat butter or soy margarine in nonstick skillet until melted. In a medium-sized mixing bowl combine 1 cup of Arrowhead Mills Multi-Grain Pancake and Waffle Mix, nutmeg, cinnamon, mashed banana, and applesauce. Add melted butter. Pour in milk or soy or vanilla-almond beverage. Beat until batter is free of lumps. For each pancake, pour 2 tablespoons batter onto a hot griddle or nonstick skillet. Turn pancake over after bubbles have disappeared from the top of the pancake and small pin openings appear all over pancake. Edges should also look cooked. Repeat until done.

12 SERVINGS
1 serving (1 pancake): 1.5 fat grams, 62 calories

Crystal's Low-Fat Chicken Caesar Salad

I don't use a scale much to watch my weight. I watch my behavior toward exercise, food, and how my clothes are fitting.

INGREDIENTS

2 fresh bundles romaine lettuce, washed and chopped

2 washed ripe tomatoes, chopped

1 washed bell pepper, chopped

½ cup grated fat-free mozzarella cheese or Soya Kaas fat-free mozzarella

½ cup nonfat garlic croutons

nonfat Caesar dressing

CHICKEN BREAST

1½ lbs. skinless, boneless chicken breast, cubed

teaspoon salt or sea salt

teaspoon poultry seasoning

teaspoon oregano

teaspoon garlic powder

SALAD

2 fresh bundles romaine

Preheat oven to 500°F. Season chicken breast with salt, poultry seasoning, oregano, and garlic powder. Bake for 3 to 4 minutes or stir-fry at high temperature. Let cool before adding to salad.

Combine salad ingredients. Top with cooled chicken and Caesar salad dressing

6 SERVINGS

1 serving (4 ounces chicken and 1 cup salad): 4 fat grams, 382 calories

Crystal's Grilled Sweet Slammin' Salmon

Restrictive eating is for those who want to imprison their mind, body and spirit.

INGREDIENTS FOR SWEET SAUCE (MARINADE)

**½ cup honey
½ cup "Tree of Life natural stone-ground mustard with herbs" (low sodium, no sugar) or regular mustard
1 teaspoon each of paprika, ground ginger, sea salt or regular salt, poultry seasoning, basil, and garlic powder**

Put ingredients in bowl and mix well, then put into Ziploc bag.

ATLANTIC SALMON

4 6-oz. 1-inch-thick salmon steaks

Add salmon to bag. Seal and marinate in refrigerator for 2 hours, occasionally turning bag.

Tell the family griller to light the grill and to wrap the grill rack with aluminum foil.

Remove salmon from bag, reserving the marinade. Place salmon on grill rack and cook for 5 to 6 minutes (basting frequently with reserved marinade) on each side or until fish flakes easily when tested with a fork.

4 SERVINGS

1 Serving (1 salmon steak): 14 fat grams, 350 calories

Put the children to bed. Dim the lights and have a candle-light dinner on the patio or deck and gaze at the moon while your special man puts on some soft jazz, gospel, or blues music. While he's putting on the music, bring out the leafy vegetables, a small baked potato, and a glass of your favorite beverage. I'll leave the dessert up to you.

Aunt Vernell's Rosemary Potatoes

Eat whole-quality foods for physical and mental satisfaction.

INGREDIENTS

    1 tablespoon rosemary
    1 tablespoon garlic powder
    1 tablespoon paprika
    ¼ teaspoon sea salt or regular salt
    1½ tablespoons extra virgin olive oil
    4 red potatoes (around 1½ pounds), washed, leaving on skin, each cut into 6 wedges

Preheat oven to 400°F.

    Combine all ingredients, including potatoes, in a large plastic Ziploc bag and seal closed. Shake well until all potatoes are coated with spices. Take potatoes from plastic bag and arrange in a single layer in a shallow roasting pan; bake at 400°F. for 35 minutes, or until potatoes are tender.

4 SERVINGS

    1 Serving (1 cup): 7 fat grams, 254 calories

Italian Turkey Sausage Spaghetti

Journal writing is my greatest source of comfort. It records my life, it helps me remember, and keeps me honest about what I eat and why.

INGREDIENTS

2 teaspoons extra virgin olive oil
1 tablespoon oregano
1 teaspoon basil
2 tablespoons fresh chopped garlic
1 cup fresh broccoli flowerets (chopped)
1 cup snow peas
1 package ground Italian turkey sausage
8 oz. of organic or regular uncooked spaghetti
2 tablespoons chopped fresh parsley

Lightly coat a large nonstick skillet with olive oil. Place over medium-high heat until hot. Add oregano, basil, garlic, broccoli, and snow peas, and sauté 3 minutes. Stir in ground Italian Turkey sausage. Cover, reduce heat, and simmer 6 minutes. Cook pasta according to package directions. Add pasta to vegetable/sausage mixture; toss well. Sprinkle with parsley and serve.

8 SERVINGS

1 serving (1 cup): 7.3 fat grams, 180 calories

Light Vegetable Lasagna

Listen to your body and know your body better than any doctor. Give thanks to God for your good health because without it you have nothing.

INGREDIENTS

4 red bell peppers cut in half lengthwise (discard seeds and membranes)
6 yellow squash, halved lengthwise and cut into 1-inch pieces
½ teaspoon sea salt or regular salt
½ teaspoon black pepper
4 garlic cloves, minced
1 large onion, chopped
1 teaspoon dried oregano
½ cup chopped fresh basil
1½ cups grated sharp provolone cheese or soy mozzarella with tofu
½ cup grated part-skim mozzarella cheese
2 cups low-fat cottage cheese
2 cups spinach leaves, chopped
9 whole-wheat or regular cooked lasagna noodles

Preheat broiler. Place pepper halves on a foil-lined baking sheet and broil 15 minutes, or until blackened. Combine oil, salt, black pepper, squash, and onion on same foil-lined baking sheet and bake for 20 minutes at 450°F. Take from oven and combine with garlic in a bowl. Decrease oven temperature to 375°F. Combine all cheeses (cottage cheese, too) with dried oregano and basil. Spread bottom of pan with 1/3 teaspoon extra virgin olive oil. Arrange 3 noodles over saucepan; top with 1 cup of cheese mix-

ture, 1 cup spinach, 4 bell-pepper halves, 2 cups vegetable mixture. Repeat layers, ending with noodles.
Cover and bake at 375°F. for 15 minutes. Uncover;
sprinkle with mozzarella cheese. Bake another 20
minutes.

10 SERVINGS

1 serving (1 medium-sized square): 10 fat grams,
277 calories

Oven Crispy Catfish

Just because I've have been cut by the thorn of a rose doesn't mean I don't want roses anymore. I'll just pick my roses with care and patience the next time around.

When choosing a catfish I like to choose one that is farm-raised. You'll find it tastes cleaner and has less fat.

INGREDIENTS

**6 Farm-raised catfish fillets, washed
(cut in half if too thick)
garlic powder
poultry seasoning
basil
oregano
thyme
paprika
white pepper**

Preheat oven to 500°F.
Season both sides of fillets with salt and spices.

Place fillets on nonstick cookie sheet and bake until crispy-brown on both sides, for a total of 25 minutes.

5 SERVINGS

1 serving (1 fillet): 6 fat grams, 180 calories

Quick Savory Sweet Potatoes

You can make a way out of no way.

INGREDIENTS

    1 Medium sweet potato, washed and cut into 4 wedges
    sprinkle of cinnamon
    sprinkle of nutmeg
    1 teaspoon soy margarine or butter
    ¼ teaspoon sea salt or regular salt
    1 teaspoon honey

Place sweet potato in microwave-safe container with a cup of water. Put in microwave and hit the potato setting (approximately 15 minutes) and let the microwave do the rest. Test the sweet potato with a fork to make sure it is ready (fork should easily go through potato). You can keep the skin of the potato on or peel it off. Mash potato and mix with other ingredients and enjoy!

1 SERVING

    (1 medium potato): 4 fat grams, 153 calories

Quick and Easy Black Beans and Rice

Accept where you are now and work toward your goal of being healthy.

INGREDIENTS

2 16-oz. cans black beans, drained
1 can nonfat chicken broth
1 bay leaf
2 teaspoons oregano
2 teaspoons sea salt or regular salt
2 cups shredded carrots
3 teaspoons lemon juice
1 large chopped onion
2 teaspoons fresh-crushed garlic
4 stalks chopped celery
2 teaspoons of hot red pepper
3 cups brown rice or basmati rice

Cook rice separately according to directions. Combine beans and all other ingredients and let come to a boil. Reduce heat and simmer for 30 minutes.

8 SERVINGS

1 serving (1 cup): 1 fat gram, 460 calories

Caribbean Chicken Stew

I love myself more than I love that extra helping of food.

INGREDIENTS

10 ounces boned and skinned chicken breast, cut into strips
1¼ cups water
1 tablespoon olive oil
2 small bunches scallions, chopped
2 teaspoons freshly chopped ginger
1 finely grated rind of lime
2 tablespoons fresh lime juice
3 tomatoes, seeded and chopped
1 teaspoon sea salt or regular salt
1 tablespoon rum
1 tablespoon light-brown sugar
1 teaspoon ground cinnamon

Put the chicken and water in a saucepan and bring to a boil, then lower to medium heat. Cook for 10 minutes or until water has evaporated and the chicken is tender. Remove from the heat and set aside. Heat the oil in a large nonstick frying pan or saucepan and stir-fry the scallions for 2 minutes. Drain the cooked chicken strips and add them to the pan. Stir-fry for 3 minutes over medium heat. Gradually add all other ingredients. Toss over the heat to warm tomatoes through and let the flavors blend together. Put into a serving dish and enjoy!

4 SERVINGS

1 serving (1 cup): 8.2 fat grams, 155 calories

TWO WEEKS OF MENUS

*I*n this section you'll find two weeks' worth of menus. These are all the foods I ate to lose weight and still continue to eat in order to keep the weight off. Since I tend to work out very early in the morning, I usually eat like a king (large portion) in the morning, eat like a queen (medium portion) at lunchtime, and eat like a pauper (small portion) at dinnertime, before 7 P.M. I also include 3 small healthy snacks throughout the day.

But I've found with new members of my workshop who have a family that the average person usually doesn't eat breakfast, or if she does, it's very little because most people eat dinner between 6 and 8 P.M. That's why the breakfast menus are light. But if you do eat like a king at breakfast, increase the portion sizes and eat.

For those of you who do *not* eat breakfast in the morning, try to eat something. This will boost your metabolism in the morning, especially if you exercise. If you exercise, then eat breakfast afterward, you will boost your metabolism a lot earlier and keep it elevated for a longer period of time. I found when members of my weight-loss workshop started to include exercise (morning or evening) in their daily life and stopped eating after 9 P.M., they tended to be hungry in the morning and started losing weight.

If you can't fit exercise into your schedule in the morning, that's okay, but find a way to fit it in sometime because that will be the key to losing weight and keeping it off. When you start to incorporate exercise you'll find that you will need breakfast in the morning.

Note that I have given you the option of eating real bacon within *reason*—2 slices—or turkey bacon. Remember not to fry your bacon. Try popping it in the oven or microwave, letting it cook at the highest temperature, and draining it on paper napkins afterward to get rid of the grease. Try to use light olive oil, canola oils, sesame oil, or Asian oil whenever possible instead of heavy lards. Remember, we're trying to get rid of the lard in our bodies. Watch your alcohol intake and use alcohol in moderation, as well as diet sodas (they still contain some forms of sugar).

Also note that I have included soy margarine and soy beverages for those who have allergies or cannot digest dairy products. I use canola mayonnaise that is low in saturated fat, and soy products and Rice Dream, which have calcium. And since I can't stand the taste of no-fat dressings, no-fat cheese and mayonnaise, I eat the real thing or soy cheese. I'd much rather have one teaspoon of something that tastes good than half a bottle of something that tastes horrible. I've also included snacks between meals because I've always snacked and I didn't want to feel deprived. Like I said before, I eat six small meals throughout the day. You should also check with your physician before making any lifestyle changes.

You'll see that I did not include any portion sizes in the menu. Not everyone can eat the same portions because their weight-loss goals are different. Personally when I see four ounces of meat or a half a cup of vegetables I immediately think "diet" and start feeling deprived, and I didn't want to go there. Remember, this is only a guide.

SERVINGS

1 slice of bread: the size of a compact-disc case.

The palm of your hand is approximately three ounces of cooked meats or fish.

The row of knuckles on your hand is approximately five ounces of cooked meats or fish.

The size of your fist is approximately the size of a medium fruit.

The size of a tennis ball is approximately one cup of cooked rice or vegetables.

The size of a half-dollar or the tips of your fingers is approximately one teaspoon.

If you cup your hand, that's approximately one ounce of peanuts, cheese, or dry cereal.

1 Milk/juice/soy milk/Rice Dream with calcium: 1 cup (try to use one-percent milk or skim milk)

Sodas/pop: 1 12-oz. can. Try to limit intake to one a day and replace the rest with water.

Wine: 1 regular 4–6oz. wine glass

Beer: 1 regular 12-oz. can or bottle (no megabottles)

Liquor: a shot glass

Try to cut red meat consumption in half and replace with baked or grilled chicken breast, turkey breast, or baked fish.

Limit the following to:

Pastas: 1 cup cooked

Rice: 1 cup cooked

Hot cereals: 1 cup cooked

Cold cereals: 1 cup

Sour cream: 1 teaspoon

Soup: 1 cup

Margarine/butter/soy margarine/cream cheese: 1 teaspoon

Maple syrup: 1 tablespoon

Dressing: 1 tablespoon

Cheese: 1 ounce

Nuts: 1 ounce

Crackers: limit 5 (15 grams), about the size of Ritz light

Graham crackers: 2

Potato chips/pretzels: 1 one-ounce bag

Popcorn: 1 three-ounce bag

Sherbet or sorbet: 1 cup

Ice cream: ½ cup

Sodium: Follow your physician's guidelines

Diabetes and hypertension patients: Follow your physician's guidelines

If you choose to eat a late-night snack, try to make it a fruit or vegetable. And, since it's preferable to eat your last snack or meal three hours before bedtime, try to stick as close to this rule as possible.

If you don't like one of the meals, don't force yourself to eat it. Replace it with one from another day's menu.

There is plenty of food to eat at meals, along with snacks throughout the day. If you can't eat the snacks because you are full, don't eat them. If you get hungry at other times of the day like I did, feel free to add another fruit or vegetable.

Remember to calculate your water intake. Divide the number of pounds you wish to lose by 25 *only* if you have 45 or more pounds to lose. If you have to lose 10 to 40 pounds, drink eight (8-ounce) glasses of water a day. Don't forget the amount of water you drink increases as you exercise and as the weather gets hot and dry. I like to squeeze fresh lemon juice into my water or put a lemon wedge in my water in the morning to help flush out my system. Go ahead and drink water like a fish. And last but not least, I've put in reminders for you to exercise—remember, this is the other component to successful permanent weight loss.

DAY 1
Exercise with Sips of Water

—

BREAKFAST:

Orange juice/milk/soy milk

Oatmeal

SNACK:

A mango

Drink water.

LUNCH:

Roast-turkey sandwich on whole-wheat bread with
tomato, romaine lettuce, 1 slice of cheese of
choice, and mustard

Mixed salad

Low-fat yogurt

Drink water.

Favorite low-calorie beverage

SNACK:

Raisins or 1 small low-fat bran muffin

Drink water.

DINNER:

Grilled skinless chicken breast

Steamed cabbage

Baked potato, small pat of butter or soy margarine with
a *little* of your favorite seasonings.

Mama's Sugar-Free Banana Pudding (See recipe
section)

Drink water.

Favorite low-calorie beverage

SNACK:

Fruit or vegetable

DAY 2:
Exercise with Sips of Water

—

BREAKFAST:

Orange

Whole-wheat toast with a trace of low-fat
  margarine/butter or soy margarine

SNACK:

Low-fat yogurt

Drink water.

LUNCH:

2 slices of thin-crust cheese pizza (Pizza Hut) or 2 slices
  of vegetable pizza, no cheese

Tomato-basil salad, balsamic vinaigrette dressing

Grapes

Skim milk/1-percent-milk or non-dairy beverage with
  calcium

Drink water.

SNACK:

1 small bag of pretzels or fruit

Drink plenty of water.

DINNER:

Crispy Catfish (See recipe section)

Broccoli

Corn on the cob

Watermelon

Drink water.

Favorite low-calorie beverage or glass of wine or a
  12-oz. beer or 1 shot glass of liquor

SNACK:

Sliced pineapple

DAY 3:
Exercise with Sips of Water

—

BREAKFAST:

   Whole-grain low-fat waffles with favorite fruit
   Maple syrup
   Drink water or herbal tea with a fresh-squeezed lemon
       wedge.

SNACK:

   Graham crackers or apple-cinnamon rice cakes
   Drink water.

LUNCH:

   Quick Savory Sweet Potato (See recipe section)
   Lean beef or Low-Fat Chicken Caesar Salad (See
       recipe section)
   Drink water.
   Favorite low-calorie beverage

SNACK:

   Low-fat tortilla chips with salsa
   Drink plenty of water.

DINNER:

   Italian Turkey Sausage Spaghetti (See recipe section)
   Spinach salad with honey-mustard dressing
   Orange sherbet
   Drink water.
   Favorite low-calorie beverage

SNACK:

   Fruit or vegetable

DAY 4:
Day off from Exercise!

~

BREAKFAST:

    Whole-wheat English muffin with thin layer of favorite
        jam
    Apple juice

SNACK:

    Apple
    Drink water.

LUNCH:

    Kelley's Tantalizing Tuna (See recipe section)
    With favorite pasta or bread or crackers
    Tossed salad with favorite dressing
    Drink water.
    Favorite low-calorie beverage

SNACK:

    Bagel with thin layer of cream cheese
    Drink water.

DINNER:

    Lean beef or shrimp pasta salad
    Steamed asparagus
    Grilled vegetables
    Basmati rice
    Honeydew melon
    Drink water.
    Favorite low-calorie beverage

SNACK:

    Fruit or vegetable

DAY 5:
Exercise with Sips of Water

—

BREAKFAST:

    Crystal's Apple-Banana Pancakes (See recipe section)
        with maple syrup
    Blueberries or strawberries

SNACK:

    Sliced apple
    Low-calorie yogurt as dip

LUNCH:

    Fresh Turkey Necks and Cabbage (See recipe section)
    Mama's Buttermilk Cornbread (See recipe section)
    Drink plenty of water.

SNACK:

    Low-fat lemon scone
    Drink water.

DINNER:

    Crystal's Grilled Sweet Slammin' Salmon (See recipe
        section)
    Aunt Vernell's Rosemary Potatoes (See recipe section)
    Sistah Woman's Naked Stir-Fried Greens without meat
        (See recipe section)
    Drink plenty of water.

SNACK:

    Raspberry sorbet

DAY 6:
Exercise with Sips of Water

—

BREAKFAST:
> Fruit juice:
> Scrambled egg whites
> Turkey bacon or real bacon
> Toasted whole-wheat bread or English muffin
> Drink plenty of water with a lemon wedge.

SNACK:
> Bagel with trace of favorite topping
> Orange slices

LUNCH:
> Fried chicken (2 pieces)
> Steamed peas, broccoli and carrots
> 1 whole-wheat roll
> Drink water.

SNACK:
> 1 Caramel rice cake
> Drink water.

DINNER:
> Quick and Easy Black Beans and Rice (See recipe
>   section)
> Tossed salad with favorite dressing
> Drink water.
> Favorite low-calorie beverage

DAY 7:
Day of Rest—No Exercise

—

BREAKFAST:

Raisin Bran with 1-percent milk or skim milk or soy
beverage
Fruit of choice

SNACK:

3 Ginger snaps

LUNCH:

Caribbean Chicken Stew (See recipe section)
Steamed vegetables
Multi-grain bagel with trace of butter or soy margarine
Fresh sliced peaches
Drink water.

DINNER:

Light Vegetable Lasagna (See recipe section)
Small piece of apple pie
Drink water.

SNACK:

Cantaloupe

DAY 8:
Exercise with Sips of Water

—

BREAKFAST:

    Honeydew melon

    Coffee or tea

SNACK:

    1 low-fat bar of Sweet Success or fruit of choice

    Drink water.

LUNCH:

    Baked swordfish

    Steamed vegetables

    Brown rice

    1 Frozen fruit bar

    Drink water.

    Favorite low-calorie beverage

SNACK:

    1 Rice pudding (1 cup) or 1 small slice of cake

DINNER:

    1 Steak kabob

    Steamed vegetables

    Wild rice

    Skim milk or wine (1 glass) or one 12-oz. can of beer

        or 1 shot glass of liquor

    Drink water.

SNACK:

    1 Whole-wheat English muffin with a trace of butter.

DAY 9:

Exercise with Sips of Water

—

BREAKFAST:

Rice Krispies or favorite hot cereal

SNACK:

Pear
Drink water.

LUNCH:

Turkey sub
Tossed salad with dressing
Nectarine
Drink water.

DINNER:

Baked flounder
Grilled vegetables
Baked potato
Low-fat yogurt
Drink water.
Favorite low-calorie beverage

SNACK:

Favorite fruit

DAY 10:
No Exercise

—

BREAKFAST:

Cornflakes or hot cereal

Banana

Drink water with lemon wedge.

SNACK:

Apple sauce (1 cup)

LUNCH:

1 Chick-Fil-A chicken nuggets 8 pieces

Tossed salad with dressing

1 Fudge brownie with nuts

Drink plenty of water.

Favorite low-calorie beverage

SNACK:

1 Bag Popcorn

Drink plenty of water.

DINNER:

Grilled whitefish with lemon

Steamed vegetables

1 Whole-wheat dinner roll with trace of butter or soy
    margarine

1 Container of low-calorie yogurt

Drink water.

Favorite low-calorie beverage

SNACK:

1 oz. Pumpkin seeds or nuts or cheese with crackers

Drink water.

DAY 11:
Exercise with Sips of Water

—

BREAKFAST:
>1 Boiled egg
>Whole-wheat toast with trace of butter
>Drink water with lemon wedge.
>Herbal tea or coffee

SNACK:
>Favorite fruit
>Drink water.

LUNCH:
>1 Lean roast-beef sandwich on multi-grain bread with
>   romaine lettuce, tomato, and trace of mayonnaise
>Tossed salad with favorite dressing
>1 Banana
>Drink water.
>Favorite low-calorie beverage

SNACK:
>Grapes

DINNER:
>Grilled or baked pork chops
>Steamed potatoes
>Green beans
>1 Frozen fruit bar
>Drink water.
>Favorite low-calorie beverage

SNACK:
>Fruit or vegetable

DAY 12:
Exercise with Sips of Water

———

BREAKFAST:

    Turkey sausage

    Whole-wheat toast

    Drink water with lemon wedge.

    Favorite low-calorie beverage

SNACK:

    1 Grapefruit

LUNCH:

    Wendy's chili

    Tossed salad with dressing

    2 Snackwell cookies

    Drink water.

    Favorite low-calorie beverage

DINNER:

    Chicken Out or Boston Market—turkey breast or
        chicken breast

    Tossed salad with dressing

    1 Whole-wheat dinner roll or dressing or macaroni and
        cheese

    Drink water.

    Favorite low-calorie beverage

    1 Large slice of angel food cake with strawberries

SNACK:

    1 small apple

DAY 13:
Exercise with Sips of Water

—

BREAKFAST:
> Favorite cereal with fruit
> Water with lemon wedge

SNACK:
> 1 Low-fat yogurt shake
> Drink water.

LUNCH:
> 1 Chicken pita with romaine lettuce, tomato and onion
>   sprouts
> Low-fat pasta salad
> Frozen yogurt
> Drink water.
> Favorite low-calorie beverage

DINNER:
> Vegetable chicken soup with brown rice
> Steamed vegetables
> 1 Bread stick
> Drink water.
> Favorite low-calorie beverage
> 1 Frozen Fudgesicle

SNACK:
> Favorite fruit or pretzels/potato chips/popcorn
> Drink plenty of water.

DAY 14:
Day of Rest—No Exercise

—

BREAKFAST:

Whole-wheat pancakes with trace of margarine/butter
or soy butter
Sliced banana or strawberries
1 Low-fat turkey sausage or two strips of bacon
Drink plenty of water.

SNACK:

Sunflower seeds or fruit
Drink water.

LUNCH:

1 Small vegetable pot pie
½ cup Grilled vegetables
Drink water.
Favorite low-calorie beverage.

SNACK:

1 Medium peach

DINNER:

Baked fish or chicken or turkey breast
Mixed raw vegetables with Dressing
1 whole-wheat dinner roll
1 Glass wine or one 12-oz. can beer or 1 shot glass of
liquor or favorite low-calorie beverage
1 Chocolate-chip cookie
Drink water.

SNACK:

Fruit or vegetable

BIBLIOGRAPHY

Avila, Patricia, *Fitness for Health and Sports.* Granite Bay. CA: Penmarin Books, 1999.

Ferrell, Pamela. *Let's Talk Hair.* Washington, D.C.: Cornrows & Co., 1996.

Fraser, Laura. *Losing It. False Hopes and Fat Profits in the Diet Industry.* New York: Plume/Penguin Group, 1998.

Fritschner, Sarah, and Michael F. Jacobson, Ph.D. *The Completely Revised and Updated Fast Food Guide,* second ed. New York: Workman Publishing Company, Inc., 1996, 1991.

Garrison, Jr., Robert, and Elizabeth Somer, *The Nutrition Desk Reference.* New Canaan, Connecticut: Keats Publishing, Inc., 1995.

Herbert, Victor, M.D. and Genell J. Subaksharpe, M.S. *Total Nutrition: The Only Guide You'll Ever Need.* New York: St. Martin's Griffin, 1995.

Hollis, Judi. *Fat Is a Family Affair.* United States of America: Hazelden, 1985.

L., Elisabeth. *Twelve Steps for Overeaters*. United States Of America: Hazelden, 1993.

Martins, Peter. *New York City Ballet Workout—Fifty Stretches and Exercises Anyone Can Do for a Strong, Graceful, and Sculpted Body*. New York: Quill/William Morrow and Company, Inc. 1997.

Nanfeldt, Suzan. *Plus Style*. New York: Plume/Penguin Group, 1996.

Neporent, Liz, with John Egan. *Crunch—A Complete Guide to Health and Fitness*. New York: Main Street Books/Doubleday, 1997.

Podjasek, Jill H. *The Ten Habits of Naturally Slim People—And How to Make Them Part of Your Life*. Lincolnwood (Chicago), Illinois, 1997.

Roth, Gennen. *Breaking Free From Compulsive Eating*. New York: Plume/Penguin Group, 1993.

Ulene, Art, M.D. *The Nutribase Guide to Fat and Cholesterol In Your Food*. New York: Avery Publishing Group, 1995.

Villarosa, Linda. *Body and Soul—The Black Women's Guide to Physical Health and Emotional Well-Being*. New York: HarperCollins Publishers, 1994.

Zerbe, Kathryn J., M. D. *The Body Betrayed—A Deeper Understanding of Women, Eating Disorders, and Treatment*. Carlsbad, CA: Gurze Books, 1995.